HEALTHY LIVING OVER 55

Since 1978 the 'Getting On' television programme has been a leader in the drive for a positive approach towards ageing. Laura Mitchell's contributions to the programme have been very much in that spirit, as her new book – which is based on the current Central Independent Television series – shows. She says it is 'not a guide to perfect bodies, just to useful ones'. Exercises, fitness and full use of one's body are important not as ends in themselves but because they allow us to go on living a full and active life.

She is frank on what you can and can't do about your skin care, including a full range of wrinkle exercises for the face. From the externals she passes to the internals of the head, with practical advice on eyesight, hearing, teeth, memory, relaxation, and sleep. She offers exercises so that you can keep your shoulders mobile (so important when getting dressed) and unfold stiff arthritic hands (vital for maintaining one's independence).

She is keen for you to re-examine how you walk, sit and stand. There is advice on balance so you can sway safely and remain effective while standing on one leg (an ingredient in many sports). She explains foolproof methods for getting in and out of chairs, cars, beds and baths, and how to use a stick if you have to. She shows how to stretch the spine, breathe properly, strengthen the heart and take positive steps against incontinence. There are sections on hypothermia, using the kitchen as a gym, safety at home, getting away from the tea-and-biscuits diet, visiting patients in hospital and being a patient yourself, convalescing and getting back to normal.

The maturity of her approach is reflected in her explanations of *how* the body works so we know *why* we should exercise in certain ways. Again she is concerned at all times to tailor her advice to the real concerns and conditions facing her own age group.

LAURA MITCHELL, MCSP, dipTP, is well-known in British physiotherapy and obstetric circles. Her physiological method for easing tension is now used worldwide. Her book about it, *Simple Relaxation*, was published in 1977 and its sequel, *Simple Movement* (written with Barbara Dale), in 1980.

HEALTHY LIVING OVER 55

'Getting On' Guide

LAURA MITCHELL

JOHN MURRAY

CENTRAL INDEPENDENT TELEVISION

This publication is based on the television series 'Getting on'
produced by Central Independent Television plc

© Laura Mitchell 1984

'Getting On' programme material © 1984 Central
Independent Television plc

First published 1984
by John Murray (Publishers) Ltd
50 Albemarle Street, London W1X 4BD
and Central Independent Television plc
Central House, Broad Street, Birmingham B1 2JP

Typeset by Inforum Ltd, Portsmouth
Printed and bound in Great Britain
by Richard Clay (The Chaucer Press), Bungay, Suffolk

British Library Cataloguing in Publication Data
Mitchell, Laura
   Healthy living over 55.
   1. Aging
   I. Title
   612'.67   QP86
   ISBN 0–7195–4112–3

Contents

Contents

Acknowledgements

I wish to thank Roger Hudson of John Murray, my publishers, for his patience and expertise in coping with oddments of writings over many months, as I successively disappeared into and escaped from hospital. I will always be grateful to the surgeons, doctors, and other hospital staff for their skill and kindness which eventually produced my complete recovery.

I am much indebted to Michael Bartlett for his meticulous drawing and redrawing of the pictures. I also wish to thank Tony Budd, my producer at Central Independent Television. He has shown so much interest and enthusiasm for my ideas in fostering the health of the over fifties. It has been a great privilege to work with him and the *Getting On* team. The literature put out by Help The Aged, Age Concern, the Health Education Council, and the Royal Society for the Prevention of Accidents has been invaluable.

So many of my friends of all ages have given me much valuable support, inspiration and comfort. I could not have undertaken the book and series at all without their aid. I hope that both programmes and book will be useful to my fellow 'over-fifties'.

The urgent need is for 'old' people to learn to fight back against hogwash, classification, put downs and rip offs which, by virtue of the passage of time alone, society writes into the roles of people who could still be young.

DR ALEX COMFORT, *A Good Age*, 1976

Director of Research, Gerontology, 1966–73, University College London. President of the British Society for Research on Ageing, 1967

Introduction

In April 1982 Age Concern, England, in association with the Department of Health and Social Security held a conference called 'Add Life to Years' at the invitation of the World Health Organisation. Later that summer the United Nations World Assembly held its first full-scale conference on 'Ageing' in Vienna. Representatives of one hundred and twenty countries took part, and drew up a world plan of action which especially stressed self-care and nutrition. This book and my contributions to the accompanying Central Independent Television series *Getting On* are particularly focussed on just this approach.

The *Getting On* series has been running since 1978, giving information and entertainment to older people fortnightly on Sunday mornings. All of us involved in the programme try to serve their needs, to stimulate and to encourage.

There are more than 10 million people aged 60 or over in Britain, more than the number of school children. Many old people are sprightly, have good health and a happy, satisfying life, but you can easily go downhill following an illness or bereavement. Then, at the other end of the scale, there are those who have entirely forgotten how to maintain movement and how to take care of their general health. You may be in great danger of further deterioration and then would need a geriatric hospital bed. In 1981, 45 per cent of all National Health Service beds were filled by people over 65 years old.

Many of these are admitted for treatment due to an acute illness or an accident. They tend to remain in hospital longer than younger patients with similar conditions, and indeed some stay for the remainder of their lives and become 'bed blockers'. If, by taking care, some of these people could remain healthy and happy in their own homes, great reductions in the waiting queues of other patients could be achieved.

I hope to encourage older people and those who look after them to cultivate body awareness and to enable them to have a more healthy and satisfying life style. Then they can continue to go out, maintain old interests, join or form new groups for sport, dancing, painting, cooking, politics, citizens' band radio, etc., and possibly be of service to others. Exercise is not an end in itself. But it can be a new beginning or a way of making sure that you go on living a full life, and enjoying it. Let me make it clear at once that I will *not* be advocating strenuous sport, exercises, jogging, yoga or isometrics; although, of course, some of you may advance to these if you so wish.

After retirement comes a wonderful opportunity to use the extra time and the accumulated experience at your disposal for the benefit of yourself and others. About two thousand years ago, Cicero wrote in his treatise on old age, 'It is not by miracles, speed or physical dexterity that great things are achieved, but by reflection, force of character and judgement: in these qualities old age is usually not only not poorer, but even richer'. We spend our lives wanting to be mature. Well, now we are, so let's make the most of it. To do this, we must keep in trim, mobile and interested in ourselves and the community, in other words, in life.

Few people, whatever their age, are in perfect health all the time, but trouble in one area need not mean overall deterioration of the whole body, or a shrinking of the personality because of forced reliance on others. Don't say 'It's my age'. Illness affects all ages.

During most of my life, I have suffered from arthritis of the spine and, in recent years, also of the hips. For the last eleven years, I have had a chronic infection of my right hip – osteomyelitis. This has meant continuous chemicotherapy, bouts of hospital, bed or using crutches. I have had four hip operations and a mastectomy for breast cancer. Yet, by looking after my general health as much as possible and by maintaining what movement was available to me, I can honestly say I have continued to enjoy life and found it full of excitement. This interest included broadcasting on radio and TV, writing three books on health, and meeting many new people who supported and treated me. Without them, I could never have stayed the course.

I am now learning to walk with an artificial hip joint on one side, which functions perfectly, and no hip joint at all on the other. But the good news, following this drastic operation, is that the infection is cured; I no longer need to clean a discharging wound daily. I now need no antibiotics or pain-killers – just patience and practice. I only mention all this to encourage others who are 'getting on' – I am now seventy-seven – never to give in to apparent calamity. There is always a way through, and there is always interest to be found along the way.

It is a surprise to some people to hear that exercise actually strengthens the heart, and that the increased activity of cells all over the body during exercise persists afterwards for some hours. Some people who specialise in looking after the elderly believe that good, fresh food and exercise are probably the most effective ways to lengthen life. Those who improve most are those who have been least active and in low general health.

The body is always trying to crumple into the position it

had in the womb, if we allow it. We have continually to prevent this by using the muscles which stretch and open out our bodies because the muscles which bend us into a bundle always tend to be the stronger. 'Prevention by movement' or 'Use it, don't lose it' must be the slogan at our age, and in any state, even when some other areas of the body may need rest. The only exception is in acute fever when the whole body requires total inactivity for a limited period.

The book is divided into areas of the body but, of course, all the body works together and is also influenced by the mind and emotions. Modern care of the body always regards the person as a whole, is 'holistic' in its approach. Faulty diet will affect every area and every working of the body. Neglect of any part harms the whole, and upgrading any part helps the health of the whole. I agree with A.C. Guyton, the brilliant American physiologist, who says in the Preface to his book *Function of the Human Body*: 'It has been my desire to demonstrate the beauty of organisation of the parts of the body, and to fit these together into an overall whole – a thinking, sensing, functioning human being capable of the immense diversity that characterises only higher forms of life.'

By swinging your arms, you strengthen the muscles and loosen the joints of your shoulders but you also increase the circulation of blood around the whole body and so strengthen your heart and breathing and even relieve strain on the veins of your legs. This is the meaning of the term 'aerobic exercise' (see p. 84). If you dance to music, you not only strengthen your legs, you also exercise your back and balance and develop your artistic qualities. Yes, everyone has these to some degree.

The more you understand, the less likely are you to insult your body by careless eating, by faulty activity, or by dangerous inactivity. My experience in using and teaching physiotherapy for forty years, is that people are very interested in the working of their own bodies, but they lack knowledge and are fascinated by careful explanation.

You will not find any remedies for actual illness here. There is already a multitude of books dealing with these. This book is a guide to *Health* – how to preserve and increase it and so be able to enjoy life. It is not a guide to perfect bodies – just useful ones.

Calendar age is not so important. Sometimes, the older members of our society are spoken of as though they were suddenly, at sixty, a different race. The 'little old grey-haired lady' is constantly brought before us, as though she is already half daft and wholly dependent. Such nonsense, as those who read this book and enjoy carrying out its objectives will prove. Not only will you prevent decay but you will add to the interest and quality of your life. This is what matters.

1

TAKE CARE OF YOUR

Skin

The biggest organ that you have is your skin and it is very active in preserving the health of your whole body. It is renewing itself all the time: the top layer is dead and several lower layers are always pushing up from the living cells below. If the top, dead skin is allowed to accumulate and is not washed and rubbed off daily, it becomes hard and thick and causes you trouble. It also smells unpleasantly. There are many nerve endings in skin which register heat and cold, shape, the texture of what it touches, hardness, softness, etc. This is why a baby puts everything into his mouth, where the skin is most sensitive. He is learning about the world he lives in and it is a vital activity, to be encouraged.

Who would think that, by washing the soles of your feet thoroughly and rubbing off thickened skin there, and by cutting your toe nails so that they don't protrude too far, you would be helping to keep your back straight? But it is true. Horny nails and thick skin on your feet interfere with feeling in the nerves of your feet and so with the reflex link between them and your back muscles (see p. 76).

HAIRS AND HEAT AND MOISTURE

Your skin has hairs growing out of it all over your body. These hairs can stand erect to trap warm air if you are getting cold. They also have little glands attached which exude an oily substance to help keep them – and, therefore, the skin – flexible. Beware of overheated rooms which dry out the skin. If you have to live in hot rooms, have bowls of water, containing flowers, and plants, to preserve the humidity. As you fill these up with water every day, you will realise how much fluid is disappearing into the air daily. Some of it comes from your skin. So use moisturiser patted into your skin daily. There are plenty to choose from.

Skin can stretch and then contract again (see p. 19). Think how stretched the skin of the abdomen is during pregnancy, and yet it usually recovers itself completely after the baby is born because of the elastic fibres in the skin. To help this elasticity, the skin likes to have suitable cream smoothed into it, as well as moisturiser – especially the hands, face and arms exposed to the weather, also the legs and feet. You should try several to see what suits your particular skin, and then use it daily.

Sweat Glands and Heat Loss

The body has a profit and loss system of heat control to keep your temperature at about 98.47° Farenheit (37°C). Part of the loss system are the sweat glands all over your body; the hands, neck, armpits, groin and soles of feet have many of these. When you are beginning to get too hot, much of your blood is automatically sent to your skin. There, the sweat glands manufacture sweat, send it to the surface and, as it is turned into vapour by the heat of your skin, you are cooled. But, of course, the salts and minerals remain on the skin and cause an unpleasant smell.

WASHING

A body may give off pints every day of so-called 'invisible sweat' and there is the 'visible sweat' as well, of which we are all conscious in hot weather. For the skin to keep the sweat glands active, the used sweat must be removed. This is why daily washing all over with plenty of soap and warm water is so important, to get rid of the sweat, as well as removing dead skin. Be sure the flannel, plastic sponge or loofah you use is absolutely fresh and clean. Have tepid rather than very hot water and never lie soaking in your bath. Dab on your body-moisturiser when you are half dry and this helps preserve the moisture in your skin. If you are having an all-over wash in a basin, have plenty of clean rinsing water. When sitting on the lavatory, this is a very sensible time to have a good wash down below. Washing is a great boost to your self-respect and morale. Body and mind are closely interwoven. Try to finish with something that smells delicious. Avoid harsh soaps and detergents; these can cause dermatitis. If necessary, wear rubber gloves to wash up.

Nails and Hair

Nails should be kept trimmed – finger nails rounded and the toe nails straight across – otherwise they may become horny and press into the sensitive skin, causing damage. Nails and hair also trap dirt and sweat and therefore should be washed often.

After middle life, because of the glandular changes in women, hair often grows around the lips and sometimes tufts protrude from the skin. There are safe ways to get rid of these ugly hairs.

1 You can use a magnifying glass to see the hairs clearly and pull them out with a pair of tweezers. This is quite harmless but, of course, has to be repeated.

2 You can use one of the several creams you can buy from

a chemist; they are very easy and safe to use if you follow the full instructions on the packet.

3 You can have the hairs removed by electrolysis. This is rather expensive, although very effective.

The colouring of the skin also goes rather crazy in later life. Instead of the colour being evenly spread over the whole skin, it collects in patches, rather like freckles, only larger, especially in the hands. Please don't waste money on so-called special creams to banish these patches. I have never known them to work and they will only disappoint you. If you develop warts on your skin, do show them to your doctor. She/he will decide whether they ought to be removed. Usually, they are quite harmless.

Vitamin D

Your skin manufactures vitamin D from the ultra-violet rays in sunlight. This is essential if your body is to be able to absorb the calcium it needs from your food. You may remember when rickets was a common complaint among children in cities and the frightful bone deformities they developed. This was due to a lack of proper exercise to divert blood supply to the bones, lack of calcium, phosphorus, and protein in the diet and a lack of vitamin D produced by sunlight on the skin. The result was that calcium and phosphorus were not deposited in their bones.

The same thing can happen at any age. As we get older, our bones can become brittle (osteoporosis) and people often break a leg when they fall. We therefore should include protein and calcium from milk, eggs, cheese, etc. in our diet (p. 92); then it can be transferred to our bones. Once again, the skin is looking after the health of the whole body.

So, how are you going to get the ultra-violet to your skin? By skin-airing whenever possible. You probably know that letting fierce sunlight shine on your skin is very bad for it, as well as drying it out. But you can get ultra-violet light without the hot rays if you choose early morning or early evening for skin-airing. Expose as much of yourself as you can to the air without getting cold. By doing this, as well as making vitamin D, you will be increasing the vigour of your skin and your general health.

Regulating Loss of Fluid

Urine made by your kidneys and moisture from your breath share with the skin the regulation of fluid content in your body. This, in turn, helps to regulate blood pressure. You are made of 60 per cent water. Blood, which is 80 per cent water, is the main transport system of the body, carrying food essentials, waste from worn-out cells, fatigue products, etc. Therefore, you should drink *daily* at least three to five pints of fluid. Home-made soup is a very useful article of diet (p. 93), providing, as it does, the fluid *and* the minerals that your body needs, as long as it is made out of fresh vegetables and a little meat, peas or beans.

As long as it gets the necessary fluid input, the body will then arrange the necessary balanced output of moisture, depending upon the weather, exercise, diet, humidity, etc., as they vary from hour to hour. Again we see how health depends on so many interrelated factors. The body does not function in compartments but in a unison of all its parts.

Elasticity

We have already discussed the necessity of preserving skin moisture (p. 16). The elasticity of skin can be much damaged if stretched too often or too much. If the elasticity is really lost, it will never recover. This is why women should always wear a supporting brassière. If you have difficulty fastening this, fasten in front and then twist the fastening to the back or try a petticoat with a built-in bra.

Some older women, who have had many children and not much post-natal care of their muscles, may have a rather pendulous abdomen. These should certainly wear a supporting, adjustable corset. They should also do all the back and tummy exercises suggested in Chapter 6. Muscle is wonderful at recovery if given a chance.

The skin of the legs can sometimes be stretched by swelling or varicose veins. There are various devices to support these areas, but these should never be used without the advice of a doctor. If too much support of the skin is given, it will lose whatever elasticity it had. Selection for each individual, therefore, matters very much. Of course, never use garters or anything tight like elastic around the legs. This encourages swelling.

There are foot and ankle movements in Chapter 5. You may rest with your legs on cushions, so that they are about twelve inches higher than your heart. Blocks under the castors at the foot of the bed are also sometimes useful.

Muscles in Skin

Some parts of the skin have muscles inserted into them. The ones in your face and neck you should use daily and they will

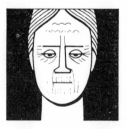

'Where the face wrinkles'

then help delay those wrinkles we all abhor. Wrinkles form in the skin at ninety degrees to the pull of the underlying muscles. So we find they are horizontal in the brow, crow's feet around the eyes and vertical on both lips. If we use the muscles attached to the skin just under these wrinkles, we stretch out the wrinkles, and by thus strengthening the muscles that support the skin, we discourage the wrinkles from forming. The best exercise of all is smiling.

FACE MOVEMENTS

You may like to use a hand-mirror to watch and enjoy your own performance.

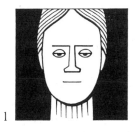

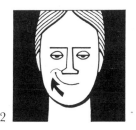

1   Brace neck muscles, pushing chin forward. Repeat twice.

2   Lift right side of mouth towards right ear and then let it slacken. Repeat twice. Lift left side of mouth towards left ear and then let it slacken. Repeat twice.

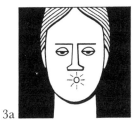

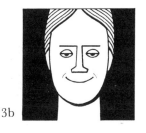

3   Purse lips and push as far forwards as possible. Draw lips backwards as far as possible, keeping lips touching. Repeat both twice.

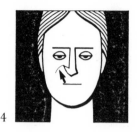

4 Raise right side of nose towards right eye; slacken it. Repeat twice. Raise left side of nose towards left eye; slacken it. Repeat twice.

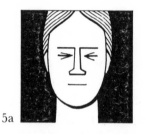

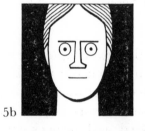

5 Squeeze eyes tightly shut. Open eyes as widely as possible. Repeat both twice.

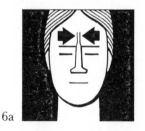

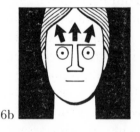

6 Draw eyebrows together and then smooth brow. Repeat twice.

2

Head and Neck

Man's Architect distinctly did ordain
The charge of Muscles, Nerves, and of the brain
Through viewless Conduits Spirits to dispense
The Springs of Motion from the Seat of Sense
DRYDEN

In the next chapter we will be considering how our environment affects our mental, emotional and physical health. In this chapter we are laying the foundation for that by looking at our sensory organs and aids, the head in which they are lodged, and the neck which supports the head. It is with the use of our eyes, ears, mouth and brain that we can see, hear, taste, smell and touch the environment, and enjoy it.

Your head weighs about 12 lbs (5kg) – that means about a stone of potatoes – and it is balanced on the smallest bone of your column of spinal bones.

Inside the seven neck bones is the rope of nerves containing all communication between your brain and your own body. They carry sensation and information from the body upwards, and orders for activity downwards. Our five senses – seeing, hearing, smelling, tasting and touching – are the means by which we know that we are alive, part of the surrounding world, and in relation with other people. The position of our heads, and the nerve and blood supply to and from this highly-developed mechanism, are of vital importance in preserving its health.

Do you realise that 15 per cent of all your blood leaving your heart on every beat, 72 times per minute, goes to your brain? The blood carries the oxygen your brain needs to function: four seconds without oxygen and you have brain damage, four minutes and you are dead. To reach your brain the blood vessels pass along a little channel in the bones of your neck (cervical spine). It therefore follows that the position of these bones affects greatly how easily the blood gets through. So we must pay attention to the position of our heads, the mobility of our joints, and the strength of our neck muscles.

NECK

Your neck is composed of seven finely made bones designed to support your head and to move it in all directions. For this purpose there are muscles running in every direction and connecting your head above with your collar bone, shoulder blade and spinal bones half way down your back. Therefore your head is very well anchored with all these muscles lying in layers, but to keep them strong it is essential to exercise them daily, otherwise your head can become very wobbly, and out of alignment with the vertebral column containing all the nerves to and from your brain. The seven bones in the neck are arranged in a forward curve and the weight of your head pressing down on it is always tending to increase this curve, and so impinge on the nerves and blood vessels within. *Never* roll your head around your neck without supporting it. You would crush the delicate bones together and make the curve greater.

Neck Exercises

Here is the safe way to exercise your neck, to keep your head in a good position and keep a good circulation of blood to and from your brain, without undue pressure on the spinal nerves. It is called a three-point pull. Sit in a chair with arms and a back tall-enough to support your head. Lay your arms on the arms of the chair so as to transfer their weight onto the chair.

Now just let the back of your head rest on the chair and stretch the top of your head towards the ceiling, keeping your eyes facing forward. At the same time pull your shoulders strongly downwards away from your ears. Do this very gently and thoroughly and you may feel your neck stretch an inch.

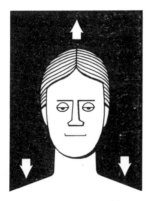

Three-point pull

Now bend your head forward, tucking your chin in. Then do exactly the opposite movement, so your nose points to the ceiling and the back of your head presses down the back of the chair.

Stretch by doing the three-point pull again, then turn your head so your nose goes over your shoulder. Stretch again and then twist in the opposite direction. Stretch again and then bend to one side so your ear comes towards your shoulder. Stretch again and bend towards the other shoulder and stretch again.

You have now used all the joints of your neck safely and fully, and strengthened its supporting muscles. These movements are safe for anyone to do and are ideal for an osteo-arthritic neck, keeping it strong and moving easily. If you have any pain down your arm or into your head, stop at once. Do the three-point pull then try carefully again. Especially do these movements if you have to wear a supporting collar. They will stop you just slumping into the collar, your neck getting stiffer and your muscles weaker. As your neck is supported by the chair you can take off your collar when you do the movements. You can also of course do them when wearing the collar (especially the three-point pull) often during the day, for a few moments at a time. Never cause pain. Anyone should be able to reach further gradually, as the muscles get stronger. When you stand, always try to balance your head with your nose facing forwards, neck stretched and your ears above your shoulders, not in front of them (see p. 74). Then you will really look your best, and keep a healthy neck, even if you do have some bony changes.

Pillows

If you have an osteo-arthritic neck, you must always take the weight of your head off it when you are sitting or in bed. Train yourself always to rest your head on the back of your chair when sitting.

In bed, whether sitting up or lying on your back, tuck a small sausage-shaped pillow into the back of your neck to preserve its forward curve. When lying on your side to go to sleep, use a feather pillow shaken to one end to form a small, firm square instead of a long oblong. Pin it tightly to make that shape. Pull it well down towards your shoulder so it fills up the space between the side of your head and the bed. It is often a comfort to stretch your arm above your head under the pillow.

YOUR FIVE SENSES

Hearing

If you find your hearing is failing, please do not just retire from human contacts, as so many people do, but ask your doctor's advice. The cause may be something quite simple, like a deposit of wax inside your ear, which can easily be syringed out. If there is some other trouble, the doctor will refer you to a specialist at a deaf clinic for further advice. Inability to hear high pitched sounds starts at about thirty years and is almost universal.

One in every three elderly people have hearing problems, and few do anything about it. They tend to disguise this even to themselves, and speak about how 'people mumble nowadays' and say they'd rather sit alone at home, than have to keep asking 'What did you say?' Tension easily builds up between the hard of hearing and their family and friends. This leads to embarrassment, often to loss of contact, even to enmity.

So what can be done? A great deal as well as expert advice.

Suppose it is decided that you need a hearing aid: you will be advised how to use it by the hearing-aid department at the hospital. Keep in touch with them and their voluntary assistants. There are so many ways they will continue to be of use to you, and will arrange frequent checks and training in the use of your hearing aid. It takes some time to learn to do so properly, so don't give up. Keep trying.

People often say their aid is no use, and stop using it, when all it may need is a new battery, some small adjustment or even washing. Ask the telephone exchange about a loud bell and the gadget to assist your hearing aid.

Aids are now so small that they are hardly noticeable. They and their maintenance are free from the N.H.S. yet less than half the deaf people have one. They are individually made to fit each person's ear, and are carefully adjusted to suit the owner's requirements. There is really no need to feel any embarrassment in wearing one. Be sure you only deal with reputable, recommended people. Swindles in deaf aids abound.

The deaf always lip-read to a certain extent even though they may wear a hearing aid. Tell anyone trying to talk to you whom you cannot hear that the worst thing they can do is to shout at you. The best thing for them is to sit opposite in a good light, speak slowly and distinctly, and re-phrase what they were saying if it is not understood. It helps if they do not smoke.

The Royal National Institute for the Deaf in London and Glasgow have a hearing advisory service which anyone can contact for help or advice.

Taste and Teeth

Please realise that your teeth are of great importance in the care of your health and in the preservation, indirectly, of your senses of taste and smell. Digestion of your food begins in your mouth and your teeth should help this process by breaking up the food. Some people cannot do this because they have neglected their teeth, perhaps need dentures, or having them, do not wear them. The food is then swallowed in lumps which cause indigestion. They are unable to eat some useful foods like wholemeal bread, apples, nuts, and they therefore have a very restricted diet. This is bad for general health, and restricts the pleasure to be got from food. Try to vary the tastes of your food from day to day and often cook something that smells delicious.

Try to preserve your own teeth as long as you live. You should see your dentist every six months so that adequate attention can be given. Even if you have neglected this, it is never too late to begin. If you wish for free N.H.S. treatment ask your local Age Concern or the D.H.S.S. for advice. Do not add to the popular idea of the ugly old person grimacing with toothless gums.

Every day brush your teeth thoroughly after meals, and use dental floss and wooden gum sticks to clear out obstinate food particles which cause decay. Any chemist can supply these very cheaply. If your gums bleed, see your dentist at once; it may mean serious trouble. Unrestricted bacteria in the mouth can cause infection there, and in the blood stream. If you need dentures please do get them fitted and then *wear them*. They keep your face in good shape. If they are not comfortable, take them back until they are, and you can eat with them quite easily. Ideally you should wash dentures after every meal, because small bits of food sticking to them can be the cause of your discomfort. Every night soak them in water with a cleanser in a covered dish. If you have to go into hospital be sure you mark your dentures, then you will know your own.

Sight

There is usually increasing difficulty in seeing objects near to you at about forty-five to fifty-five years of age. This is completely natural and happens to everyone. The lens of the eye gets harder as we grow older. Suitable spectacles, ordered by an optician is the answer. You can get a pamphlet about N.H.S. glasses from your doctor, or the social services. There is now a large variety of lenses made to suit the individual; glass lens, plastic lens, bifocals, trifocals, etc. Beware of bifocals on stairs or going up and down pavement kerbs.

It is usual to have a check-up with your optician every two years to see if your spectacle lenses need changing. This is quite often necessary, as the natural hardening process of the lens of the eyes progresses. This examination by the optician is free under the N.H.S. and you get the necessary new lenses at reduced rates. When your eyes are tested for sight the optician will also examine the health of your eyes. This is something quite different and depends on your general health. Healthy eyes do not deteriorate, except for the thickening of the lens which is purely mechanical.

Often people do not realise they are losing their sight until they find they are dropping things or stumbling dangerously on steps. Do not let yourself withdraw from everyone else, or be tempted to buy a magnifier which may not suit your eyes. Get proper advice and then do all you can to help yourself see better.

Don't try to 'save' your sight – use it. Brighten your home with light colours, and contrasting light and dark shades. In the kitchen, workroom or bathroom, use fluorescent tubes which give better light, are cheaper to run, and last much longer than ordinary light bulbs. This makes them worth the extra initial cost. Be sure your windows, net curtains, lamp shades and bulbs are sparkling clean and always sit so that you have the daylight or artificial light directed onto your work or reading. An Anglepoise lamp is a tremendous help.

Take care of your spectacles, clean them thoroughly each time you use them. Never lay them down with the glasses touching anything. This often causes scratches which distort your vision. Put them in their case whenever possible, or hang them around your neck on the special cord made for the purpose.

It is useful to have a list in very large print of all emergency phone numbers beside the telephone, so that you can quickly read them without having to find your glasses. Of course large print library books are a great pleasure.

In the kitchen and dining room use colour contrasts to help you see things. Put coloured foods like tomatoes on white plates or mats and white food like potatoes on coloured. Have a chopping board with two different coloured sides and use the dark side for white onions, the light side for red meat etc., so you chop them instead of your fingers. Use strong-coloured china from which to eat and drink, or if what you have is white, put it on a brightly-coloured cloth or on mats. Red and yellow are splendid glistening colours.

Try to find out if there is a branch of the Partially Sighted Society in your neighbourhood. Join it, and you will get much assistance from understanding people.

EYE EXERCISES

Some eyes have weak muscles controlling the movement of the eyeball. Ask your optician if this is so in your case and what eye exercises you should do. Here are safe general eye exercises.

Look Up. Look Down. Repeat 4 times. Close eyes.

Look Right. Look Left. Repeat 4 times. Close eyes.

Look up to right then down to left. Repeat. Close eyes.

Look up to left then down to right. Repeat. Close eyes.

Look slowly in a circle from left to right. Close eyes.

Look slowly in a circle from right to left. Close eyes.

Rest with eyes closed. A handkerchief put in ice-cold water and then wrung out is very comforting, draped across forehead and eyes.

Touch

Compared to the other parts of your body your hands and mouth have the largest area of your brain devoted to registering sensation in them, so please appreciate and use this sensitivity as much as you can. Develop it daily with some constructive work with your hands, which you enjoy. Try sewing, knitting, carpentry, painting, flower arranging, making a collage picture choosing various textures, gardening, baking. I know one gentleman who discovered the joys of bread making when he was over sixty. Making soft toys is another pleasurable occupation with a satisfying end product.

Every day wash something so that your hands are in warm soapy water, and then plenty of clean rinsing water. This has a primitive benign effect on our nervous systems. Try giving some soothing massage to a member of your family, using a fragrant powder or oil as a lubricant. If you keep some animal be sure you groom it every day. Both of you will enjoy the contact and the result. (See chapter 4 for more about your wonderful fingers and thumbs.)

3

Mind, Memory and Emotions

> It is notorious that the memory strengthens as you lay
> burdens upon it, and becomes trustworthy as you trust it.
> DE QUINCEY, *Confessions of an Opium Eater*

Your most precious possession in your body is your brain. Therefore, the most important ingredient for keeping your general health up to standard is to keep your brain active.

On Christmas Day 1982, the BBC had its church bells programme at 9 a.m. introduced by a man aged ninety-one, who had just had a book published on the subject. The Rev. W. Keble Martin is another example of a man over ninety who published a book. His was the *Concise British Flora* with his own coloured illustrations and it became a best seller. Catherine Bramwell-Booth, grand-daughter of the founder of the Salvation Army, published her autobiography in 1983 when she was a hundred. In the same year, Madge Sharples was the oldest woman in the London Marathon at the age of sixty-six, having started running at sixty-two to get fit before a trek to Mount Everest. Kenneth Clark was sixty-six when he gave his famous *Civilisation* series on television.

Perhaps you have an interest you could start making notes about – for an article for your local newspaper or for a book? Perhaps you would like to take a new, pleasant job, full- or part-time, or organise local groups for theatre-going, travel, bulk buying, etc.?

The brain does not get tired, but it does get bored, and it is vital to give your brain new ideas daily. Do you have the same routine every day? Then vary it. Yes, I know it takes some thinking out, but it is just this thinking that keeps your brain alive: a different newspaper, a new friend to tea, a variation of your usual meal, a new route to the shops. Solve crosswords, puzzles, get books from the library about exotic lands and different cultures. Get interested in some new subject and ask your librarian for all the information about it. Remember: 'Absence of occupation is not rest. A mind quite vacant is a mind distressed' (Cowper).

If you want to feel stimulated into pride in being human, read *The Ascent of Man* by J. Bronowski (see booklist, p. 117) and then you will certainly want to continue to nurture all your human gifts: physical, emotional, artistic and spiritual. No animal and certainly no computer can compare with *you*. Be proud of your rich human heritage and go on developing it.

Have you spoken lately to some of the younger generation and taken an interest in their activities? Do you have something living to care for? Dog, cat, budgerigar, fish, racing pigeons, geraniums, orchids – there's so much to choose from. I know one happy lady who has a devoted guinea-pig and one who has an equally happy duck!

MEMORY

Many older people say they are losing their memory. This is simply *not true*. I heard a delightful reply from a brain specialist to a lady who, complaining her memory was failing said, 'I suppose it's to be expected at my age, I'm sixty'. The specialist retorted 'If you go into any kindergarten school at lunchtime, you will find the children have forgotten all manner of things, from anoraks to balls and bats. You don't hear the children saying "Oh dear, my memory's

going, I suppose it's to be expected at five years old".'
Memory depends on *interest* not *age*. Never use that doom-laden expression "It's my age" as a reason for any kind of health or behaviour change. Health and recuperation can be achieved at any age. Widen your interests all your life, and your brain will keep active. Everyone forgets some things sometime. That is normal, so don't worry about it.

Another myth about memory is that old people remember only their early life, and have no memory for the present. The answer is that early events are polished in the brain by repetition and distance always makes us remember happy times. Often old people find their present life dull and uneventful, so they fall into the habit of forgetting. Again it comes back to *interest*. Put interest into all you do all day long and then you will have a good memory for the past *and* the present. If you are particularly interested in the social history of your lifetime you may like to join a most popular group called 'History in Action'. They visit schools and share their own interest in the past with the children.

If you like, there are a few games that you can play to train your memory. First, there is the old children's game. You select many small objects of differing shape and colour, and cover them with a cloth. Then the cloth is removed, and you look at them for only one minute, when they are again covered. You then have to write down a list of as many objects as you can remember in one minute.

There are ways of helping you to remember lists. These are *Linking*, *Exaggeration* and *Keywords*. Like your mind, the memory faculty depends upon interest and amusement so if you have a list of shopping to memorise link the words with exaggerated and amusing keywords into a story. Suppose you have a list of flour, elastic and tomatoes to buy, you might think of being given a bunch of white flowers with red balls attached by strings that bounce up and down.

Be as absurd as you can and incorporate movement, smell or vision i.e: your senses as well as similarities. Memory likes fun. The right side of your fore-brain is the site of imagination and the left side controls logic. Try to use both every day in as many ways as possible. Remember also, if you are studying, that the maximum attention time is from about five to forty minutes, depending upon interest. You then need a short rest, for five or ten minutes. So going to make that cup of coffee is not a waste of time.

Sometimes, of course, there can be illness of the brain as of any other part of the body. Your doctor can tell the difference between mental degeneration and mere lack of use. Senility in the *active* old is very rare.

WORRY, RELAXATION, SLEEP

Worry is fatal to real brain activity. When you have some worrying aspect of your life – and who has not if you are living a full life with many human contacts – solve the problem as far as you are able at the moment. Do what you can immediately, then turn the rest of the problem over to your subconscious mind to deal with. 'Sleep on it' is a good rule. Then, having 'consulted your pillow', try and solve another bit, and so on. If you are interested in the workings of the subconscious, try reading the books of Carl Jung.

The most unhealthy, unhelpful thing is to go on gnawing away at a problem, like a dog with a bone, and *doing nothing*. I suppose this is really part of the self-discipline we all need to be happy. Above all do discuss your difficulties with someone else. This is essential, so try not to be too shy to do so, because you are not alone in making mistakes or having difficulties. This is universal.

The mind is capable of holding one thought at a time, but it can switch from one thought to another interminably. If these thoughts are unhappy then we may get into a state of stress from which it is difficult to recover. Stress causes an increase of glandular output in the pituitary gland in the brain, in the thyroid gland in the neck, and in the adrenal glands above the kidneys. This in turn increases blood pressure, puts up the heart beat, causes the muscles that prepare us for fighting or running to go into action and cause sweating. Less blood goes to our digestive organs because so much has gone to the fighting muscles. All this is extremely tiring and can become dangerous if allowed to build up often.

If you find yourself in this state the first thing to do is to consider what is now called your Life Style. This means reviewing diet, sleep, amount of activity, amount of enjoyment every day, friends, hobbies, responsibilities, pets, reading, radio and television, clothing, heating, holidays, satisfaction at work or at home. All these together, if properly balanced, make for a happy stress-free life. Please seriously consider the list I have suggested and see how satisfactory you think your life style is. This is just as important, if not more so, than the method of physiological relaxation (my own Mitchell method) which I explain briefly in the following paragraphs. When you have reviewed and re-established a happy life style, and when the body tension has been relieved by relaxation, you will find your mental tension will disappear.

Remember the power of our subconscious mind is very great in its influence on our whole being. If we harbour negative emotions of envy, jealousy, resentment of past injustice, and so on, we damage our whole personalities. If we fill our conscious minds with wholesome, creative, happy thoughts and actions, refining our five senses, this permeates through and cleans up our subconscious. Then there is no room for ugly self-pity or self-deprecating dismal thoughts, or miserable inactivity.

Position of Stress

I have said that in stress the body goes into a fighting position. Probably you will recognise it, having felt it in yourself or seen it in others. This is what happens: the shoulders are raised, the arms bend up across the body, the hands clench. If sitting, the legs cross and the top foot moves up and down, or stays fixedly upward, or may wind around the other leg. If standing, you want to walk about. The body and head come forward and the breathing is either quick and shallow, or held so that you feel breathless and gasp. The diaphragm may go into spasm (cramp).

Mitchell Method of Relaxation to Relieve Stress

(This method is fully explained in *Simple Relaxation* by Laura Mitchell.)
Lie on the floor with one pillow under your head. If you prefer, sit in a chair with a back tall enough to rest your head and with arms that you can rest your arms on. If you are in bed take either of these positions. Any other position you prefer is possible, once you have practised the method.

You do not need absolute quiet for this method; have the lights on, have the room comfortably warm and do not have music as you are going to concentrate on the position of your limbs. You will develop body awareness so that in the future if, at any time, you adopt the positions of stress, you will recognise what you are doing, and will be able to get rid of them by changing very slightly your limb positions. This you must be able to do in normal everyday circumstances.

We are going to apply the physiological rules that always govern all the working of muscles in the body. In this way it is very easy to make the tense muscles let go. Here are the rules, based on the cardinal law that 'the brain knows no muscle work, only movement'.

1 You tell yourself to make a movement and the muscle work will automatically happen e.g. hop, skip, jump are three different movements. Once you have practised these you can repeat them at any time. Parts of your spinal cord and brain have learned the muscle work and the pattern is lodged in your brain. You can easily repeat it by giving yourself the order 'hop' or 'skip' or 'jump'.

2 If any group of muscles which cause a movement contracts, the opposite group will let go, i.e. relax. I have worked out what movement to tell yourself to do, so that you will cause relaxation in the tense groups.

3 You never say 'Relax'. It means nothing. You say 'Stop' when you have changed the position so you stop doing the movement. That part of your body then remains in the selected position.

4 You then very carefully recognise the pressures on your skin and the exact position of joints moved. This is very easy as these sensations go directly to the conscious brain. Never attempt to feel muscle sensation as this does not directly reach the conscious brain; it reaches the spinal cord and the lower brain. As these millions of messages of comfort flow into the brain, all the signs of stress disappear.

Now are you ready to give yourself the orders to obtain relaxation? They are very small, deliberate, adjusting movements, and you must concentrate on each as you do it, and feel what is happening. The sequence of orders is:

1 arms
2 legs
3 body
4 head
5 breathing
6 face
7 mind.

The orders in each joint are
1 move and feel
2 STOP
3 feel

ARMS

● Shoulders

Order: Pull your shoulders towards your feet.
Stop
Result: Feel your shoulders are further away from your ears.
Your neck will feel longer.

● Elbows

Order: Keep the arms on the support and push your elbows
out from body and open them slightly.
Stop
Result: Feel your upper arms away from your body and the
wide angle at your elbows. The weight of both arms should
be resting on floor, chair-arms, or pillows. Feel the exact
joint positions, and the pressure of the weight of your arms
on your skin.

● Hands

Order: Stretch your fingers and thumbs long. They fall onto
support.
Stop
Result: Feel your fingers and thumbs stretched out, separated, and touching support, nails on top. Especially feel your
heavy separated thumbs.

LEGS

● Hips

Order: Turn your hips outwards.
Stop
Result: Feel your thighs rolled outwards. Knee caps face
outwards.

- Knees

Order: Move slightly until comfortable if you wish.
Stop
Result: Feel the resulting comfort in your knees.

- Feet

Order: Push your feet away from your face, bending at the ankle.
Stop
Result: Feel your dangling heavy feet.

BODY

Order: Push your body into the support.
Stop
Result: Feel the contact of your body on the support.

HEAD

Order: Push your head into the support.
Stop
Result: Feel the contact of your head on the support and pressure on the pillow.

BREATHING

Choose rate but try to keep it slow. *Breathe in gently.* Expand the area in front above the waist, and between the angles of the ribcage; raise your lower ribs upwards and outwards like the wings of a bird. Then *breathe out gently.* Feel your ribs fall downwards and inwards. Repeat once or at most twice.

FACE

- Jaw

Order: Drag your jaw downwards.
Stop
Result: Feel your separated teeth, heavy jaw, and loose lips, especially your lips gently touching each other.

- Tongue

Order: Press your tongue downwards in your mouth.
Stop
Result: Feel your tongue touching your lower teeth.

- Eyes

Order: Close your eyes
Stop
Result: Feel your upper lids resting gently over your eyes, without any screwing up around the eyes. Enjoy the darkness.

- Forehead

Order: Begin above eyebrows and think of smoothing gently up into your hair, over the top of your head and down the back of your neck.
Stop
Result: Feel your hair move in the same direction.

MIND

Order: Either repeat the above sequence around the body, possibly more quickly. *Or* choose some subject which you will enjoy thinking about, and which has a sequence (song, prayer, poem, multiplication table, etc.). *Or* relive some past personal happy occasion. Let the mind play over these thoughts effortlessly, just to keep it occupied.

RETURN TO FULL ACTIVITY

Always stretch limbs and body in all directions and yawn. Do not hurry. Sit up slowly and wait for a minute or two before standing up.

Sleep

Sleep can be a difficulty at any age, either to get to sleep when you go to bed, or often when you awake fully conscious in the middle of the night. Another difficulty that affects the old is that they find they sleep during the day and remain awake, with a wish to be active, during the night.

This last is fairly easy to cure. It is rather obvious but few people with this problem take the trouble to solve it. The solution is to keep yourself so busy during the day that you have no time for cat naps. Reconsider your midday meal. It may be better for you to have the heavier meal in the evening, and the lighter snack at lunch time, followed by black coffee. Then immediately go out to do shopping or a walk to visit friends or to exercise the dog – and incidentally yourself.

It is essential to plan your day's meals and activity. You will already have learned whether you sleep better fasting or with a full tummy. Whichever it is, make this your routine. Then make your evening conducive to sleep. Again you must follow your own preference, some people find a walk helpful, others television, reading or laying the breakfast and perhaps preparing vegetables for next day. Think it out, but it must not be too exciting.

Then see your bedroom is the right temperature. It is no use going from a warm sitting room to an icy bedroom. Beware of half-open windows blowing a draught onto your neck (see p.   ). In winter all windows should be opened to air the bedroom in the morning for half an hour, then kept firmly shut. Woollen bedsocks are a great comfort as is a shawl to put over your head and to tuck around your neck. In summer try to wear cotton night-clothes or none at all.

Be sure you empty your bladder last thing before getting into bed and then, when you are comfortable, go through the

Mitchell method of relaxation (pp. 39–42) and finally swamp your mind with thoughts of past happy experiences. The idea is to have some easy thoughts that won't keep you awake, and which prevent you thinking up worries.

If you wake in the middle of the night, try the same routine. Get up and empty your bladder, never waste time tossing and turning and wondering what to do. Then either cool your bed or warm it up, whichever is necessary. Fetch a little something to eat – or have a tin of biscuits beside your bed. Eat whatever you choose in your comfortable bed. If you like, read a little of a very gentle kind of book, and then settle into the relaxation regime, forcing yourself by boredom to go back to sleep.

In other words you take charge of the situation and plan for it. You don't just lie there wide awake and miserable, or worse still, prowling around the house disturbing everyone else.

INDEPENDENCE

Overprotection by family or friends is one of the greatest hazards of ageing. To be treated as though you were incapable of thought or decision, and discussed over your head is most enervating. You have become a non-person. *Do not allow it.* Take your rightful place and insist on making your own decisions. Dr Alex Comfort writes 'Wasting over 16 per cent of the population doesn't seem to be in anyone's interest, especially since everyone eventually joins that 16 per cent.' Beg, borrow or even buy his book *A Good Age* if you want to appreciate the real values of ageing.

Explain to your relatives that you prefer to order your own life, even if there is some risk attached. 'Suppose you fall' they may say – well anyone can fall, and you are taking care to improve your muscle power and balance so you are less likely to do so than most. Sometimes families overprotect from a sense of guilt, but if you make it clear that it is your wish and that you have taken on the responsibility, this should expel any guilty feelings they may have.

Practise saying 'I can manage, thank you'. I have found this a magic phrase when faced with the over-officious person. Said quietly and with determination there is no answer. Do not allow strangers to use over-familiar names to you like your first name or 'Granny' or 'Old Boy'. Insist on your proper name. Over-protection leads to all kinds of unnecessary decadence in the protected person and often, eventually, to the dreaded geriatric ward. It is up to you to stop the rot as early as possible. The active exercise you take fending for yourself is an absolute essential in keeping your brain alert because it speeds the supply of blood passing through your brain, so you can think quickly.

LIVING ALONE

We, who live alone, must realise it is unnatural. Loving relationships are an essential part of human life, indeed of all life among the higher animals. When older people are left alone by the death of a spouse, or children leaving home, or even by previous choice in life, it is essential to appreciate that to live alone is very debilitating. Emotionally we depend greatly on mental and physical contact with others. The latter may mean everything from a full sexual relationship all through life, to an arm around the shoulder or holding a hand. Is not the greatest punishment in prison that of solitary confinement? If, for any reason you find yourself living alone, take stock of the situation, don't just sit and let misery overwhelm you, especially if, at the same time, you are disabled or ill in a way that makes going outside difficult.

Have you considered having a bird or animal to share

your home? It is known that solitary people who do so live longer than those who do not.

Cherish your friends of all ages, take an interest in their doings, and you will soon find they have much to offer you that you can enjoy together. Swop your miseries, mistakes, jokes and enjoyments in an honest, straightforward way. Share your burdens and pleasures. I have given a set of my front door keys to three neighbouring families. This makes access easy for them and is a comfort to me.

One of the dangers of living alone is too much radio or television. I have known people to whom soap opera characters were more important than real people. There is plenty to enjoy in radio and television for entertainment and information, but its danger is that it is all one way. You do not contribute, and anyone who is merely a spectator of life is not really alive.

As we all grow older we must maintain our vital, dangerous contact with other humans. It may mean hurt feelings, disappointments even rows, but it is life. Mixed with these negative possibilities are all the loving contacts, the hugs and kisses of children and proved relationships, and the interest of meeting new people and ideas. As Professor Guntrip says in his book *Your Mind and Your Health* 'The worst evil to which human beings can be subjected is to find themselves mentally alone, unwanted, unvalued, unrecognised, and living in a vacuum of personal relationships.'

So make your home a place that is easy to visit – never mind if it is not in apple pie order; what people enjoy is a welcome and sharing talk. The important word is *sharing*. Human relationships can be exciting as long as you live, if you keep an interest in others.

4

TAKE CARE OF YOUR

Shoulders, Arms and Hands

You probably know the famous painting by Michelangelo on the ceiling of the Sistine chapel in the Vatican, perhaps from the introductory sequence of the television arts programme *The South Bank Show*. In the centre there is the figure of God leaning forward and stretching out His arm to the figure of man whom He has just created. Each is holding out a forefinger to the other. They do not quite touch, but God's dominant right hand is obviously meant to be conveying power to the man who passively receives it through his left hand. This is an overwhelming image of the importance of man's arm and hand, all the more telling for us when we remember that Michelangelo was still sculpting marble five days before his death, in his ninetieth year.

Each of your arms is about the same weight as your head, about 12 lbs (5kg). This hefty weight is only tethered onto your body by the muscles surrounding the shoulder joints. These muscles therefore have to be very strong especially as the joints are very loose – so loose that you can pull the arm out of its socket about two inches without doing any harm. But never lift a child by his arm or hand. You could easily dislocate the shoulder by the child's body pulling downwards, while you pull the arm in the opposite direction, upwards.

Older people often sit with their arms folded or wrapped across their front because the weight of the arms is too much for the weak muscles around the shoulders. The muscles, having no work to do, get weaker and weaker while the joints probably get very stiff. A vicious circle is set up:

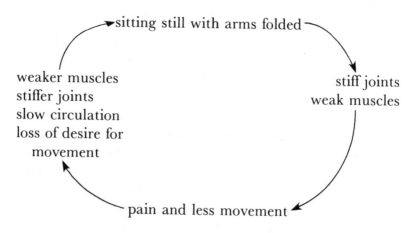

The only way out is by gentle, easy but thorough movements of the shoulders and arms gradually increasing in strength.

If you can't use your shoulders you can't use your hands, because your shoulders are there to direct your hands towards where they want to go, washing, dressing, gardening etc. Equally if for any reason you can't use one hand – perhaps following a Colles' fracture or a burn – both alas far too common – then your shoulder on that side will tend to get stiff and weak through lack of use. Be sure to keep the shoulder moving even if your wrist or hand is splinted or bandaged.

SHOULDER MOVEMENTS

The movements of your actual shoulder joint are limited to the level of your shoulder. Here is a list of those movements (begin standing, with your arm by your side):

Exact opposites	across your chest. outwards and backwards.
Exact opposites	in to the side. out sideways to shoulder level.
Exact opposites	turned inwards ie the hand and arm turns inward. turned outward ie the hand and arm turns outward.

Of course when using your arm to direct your hand in daily living these movements are all mixed. But to keep the shoulders strong and mobile you should do these movements separately and as strongly as possible. It works best if you perform the two opposite movements alternately. Move your arms one at a time or both at the same time, just as you wish. Try to keep the movements easy and rhythmic as this is much more enjoyable than stiff exercises. Think of them as movements in the dance sense, not as PT exercises or drills. If you want stronger work for the muscles, hold something like a tin of beans in your hand as you move the arm. Choose your own timing. Use music if you wish or sing as you move.

Movements above the Shoulder Level

This allows the widest movement of your hand and it is therefore the most useful. While muscles steady the arm into the shoulder joint, the shoulder blade swings around the chest and gliding movements between it and your collar bone direct your arm upwards. You are moving the shoulder blade fully when your upper arm touches your ear. Be sure you do just that.

You can do all this standing or sitting or even in bed if necessary. Of course if you stand up, you will sway about as you swing your arms, and you will be exercising your back and legs as well as your sense of balance. All this is good, if you can do it comfortably, but if your shoulders really need a lot of attention, do the movements sitting, so that all your concentration can be given to them.

If one arm is weaker or stiffer than the other, try grasping a walking stick with both hands like this:

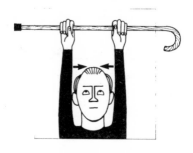

The stronger arm will help the weaker one but both must do their share. Having got both hands holding the stick, lift it straight up above your head, then lower it down to either side, and twist it about, always raising it high in between each movement. Rest as often as you like. Remember, you haven't used the muscles and joints fully unless the sides of your arms touch your ears from time to time. After your bath or shower hold the towel with a hand at each end, and use it vigorously to dry your whole body, as you exercise your arms and shoulders.

One more thing. Because the long arm bone at its top end has a knob on it, you have to twist your arm outwards before you can get the knob past the edge of your shoulder blade when lifting up your arm. You are unaware of this but often people can't raise their arms fully because the muscles that turn their arms outwards are weak. So here are two further things to do. Hang your arms down by your sides. Vigorously twist your arms inwards and outwards, especially turning outwards. You will feel the movement in your shoulder joints. When you are stronger grasp a tin of food of suitable weight in either hand as extra resistance. Later on try the exercise in the picture below which is even stronger as you are holding up the weight of your arms all the time.

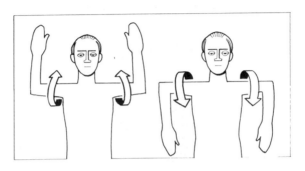

It is very important to keep on washing, dressing and undressing yourself. Strong shoulders will keep you independent. Friends and relations may find it quicker to slip on your clothing, than leave you to wrestle with it. Don't let them. Be determined always to do these things for yourself and indeed to get quicker and better at them. If you do the movements I have suggested this will help you. Later add some 'vertical press-ups'. Place your hands flat on a wall, lean your body towards the wall, then straighten your arms by pressing against the wall to push your body outwards. This strengthens the muscles that spin your shoulder blades around your chest wall. (See illustration on following page.)

Finally, avoid sitting with your arms close to your side, and your hands clasped in front. When sitting, put your arms onto the arms of the chair and have your head resting back. Swing your arms as you walk. If you have to use sticks then sometimes stand without them, lean against a table if you must, and swing your arms above your head vigorously.

You could also try watching television with your hands behind your head.

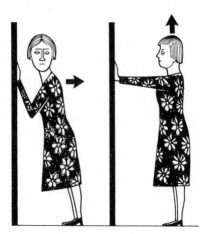

The vertical press-up

ELBOWS

The elbow is a much simpler joint. It only moves in two directions: to bend up and straighten out. So we have just two sets of muscles to strengthen around the elbow – those that bend it up and those that straighten it out. We tend to use the first lot more when eating, lifting, so it is extension that you should practise, especially the final straightening. Stretch out quickly and strongly and then hold your arm straight for a moment.

When straight this is a very firm joint. We should really use it straight when carrying shopping or a suitcase. This saves the muscle strain which happens if we carry a load on a slightly bent elbow.

THE FOREARM

It is difficult to believe that there are actually *three* moveable joints here. When your elbow is bent it is by movement in these three joints that you turn your hand over to place the palm downwards or upwards, or, most usefully, in the midway position, when your elbow is bent at a right angle. There are therefore muscles all around the forearm to control these movements, and so to control the position of your hand. A steady hand is very necessary when using the fingers and thumbs and these muscles, controlling exactly in which direction the hand is facing, hold the key.

You also use these muscles to wring clothes, to turn a door handle, or a screwdriver where the elbow is bent. When dressing, these joints are used all the time, as anyone who has had their lower arm in plaster knows. If you are unfortunate enough to suffer this, when the splint is removed be sure you work at these movements thoroughly. I have a friend now aged ninety-three who broke both her wrists in her eighties in two different falls. She persevered with movements, and still does all her own cleaning and cooking without any pain.

Everybody, I think, knows the biceps, the big muscle in front of the upper arm. It stands out like a huge sausage when you bend up the elbow with something heavy in your hand. The biceps is also the main muscle to turn your hand palm upwards (supination) so elbow bending movements, which you have already practised, will also help you to turn your palm upwards.

Movements

1 Do always wring out your face flannel very strongly, grasping it each way twice a day when you wash.

2 Tuck your elbow into your side, then hold something with a bit of weight to it in your hand and turn it quickly each way, so that the back of your hand is alternately upwards and downwards.

3 Here is a fun exercise you can do to strengthen these muscles. Clasp the fingers of each hand and resist turn.

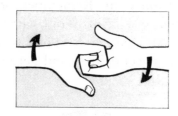

THE WRIST

The wrist bends the hand forwards about ninety degrees and extends it backwards only half as far. It also moves the hand from side to side. Again, as in the shoulder, the whole purpose of having a wrist is so that you can use your hands freely and exactly. The muscles controlling movements at the wrist lie on the front and back of the forearm. There are so many of them that they lie in layers rather like sardines in a tin. You can feel the tendons all around your wrist.

Just beyond your wrist joint in the hand there are two rows of little irregularly shaped bones. In each row there are, in fact, four bones which fit so closely into each other, just like jig-saw puzzle pieces, that across the back of the hand they feel like a smooth curve. It is actually the gliding movement between them that gives the apparently free movement of the wrist; especially is this true of the bending of the hand forward (flexion).

Some of the tendons of the muscles governing these movements only move the wrist and some reach the bones of the fingers so when you strengthen your wrist by using all these muscles, you are also strengthening your hands. If you have a so-called 'weak wrist' please do not wear one of those leather straps, which are said to 'support' it – in fact they prevent the muscles working properly and so weaken it.

People often drop things, like hot tea, over themselves simply because they have allowed the muscles of the wrist and fingers to become weak. Remember the first aid for any burn. Place the part in a basin of cold water or cover it with a towel dripping with cold water. Then treat for shock: i.e. rest, warmth, hot sweet drinks, and get help.

Movements at the Wrist

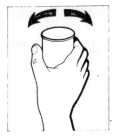

1 Take a weight in your hand. Tuck your bent elbow into your side and with your little finger towards the floor, bend and extend as often as you wish and as far as you can.

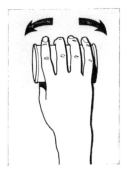

2 Turn the hand with the thumb towards the floor and move the hand to either side. Do all these movements very

slowly, strongly and carefully. Do not bang joints about — they are delicately made and are easily damaged by coarse movements.

3 You can also play that old power game facing a friend each with an elbow on the table, with hands clasped and each trying to bend his partner's hand backwards. It is quite an amusing battle if you choose someone with strength about equal to your own.

FINGERS AND THUMBS

Your fingers and thumbs are the cleverest part of your body and have the largest proportion of your brain both to receive sensation and to order movements (see p. 32, *Simple Movement* by Laura Mitchell and Barbara Dale). Some people let these wonderful instruments become practically useless through neglect.

Let us consider what your fingers and thumbs ought to be able to do.

Finger Movements

Fingers will extend to become long and straight. They will bend up so that the tips touch the cushions of flesh in the palm where the fingers join it. They can also bend down to touch the cushion of flesh at the base of the palm where it joins the wrist. If you do these two movements by way of exercise you have used the two different muscles that are situated in the forearm and which make the fingers grasp and hold anything. Extend fully between each bending.

Because you usually arrange the fingers suitably around any object that you are holding, you have four little muscles in your hand which separate each finger. You also have four which draw them close together. You can practise using these with the aid of an elastic band around the fingers moving sideways (see 1 below). Now there are four little muscles more which bend up the knuckles and at the same time straighten out the fingers. You strengthen these essential muscles by doing their own movement in the air (see 2 below).

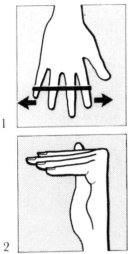

It is because you have these very small restraining muscles around the bigger tendons controlling your fingers that you can do exact work like sewing, typing, playing the piano, and other musical instruments and so on. This is why you have developed such a big section of your brain to order intricate movements and to feel the result from the joints.

Because these muscles are so small and sensitive they easily waste away to nothing if you don't keep them in use. People – especially those with any deformity in their fingers like arthritis – who sit with their hands folded up will eventually find they aren't able to do anything else. As the muscles weaken so the joints stiffen, and you can end up with completely useless hands. The hands also tend to get into weird shapes which are an embarrassment. The answer is

always *prevention by movement* – slow, rhythmic, gentle, movements for *Range* and *Power*. Now the muscle that is your real
friend in preventing these horrors is the big muscle from the
back of the forearm which ends in all the small distant bones
of the fingers, via eight tendons fixing into them. This
straightens out the fingers and extends the knuckles. As it is
put into use you frequently can see cramped hands begin to
undo themselves, to the great comfort of their owner. If you
can open your fingers out you can then arrange them suitably around an object, like a beer mug or the handle of a cup.
The small muscles of the hand assist in all this.

As I said in the Introduction, practically all the muscles,
all over our bodies, which bend us inwards tend to be
stronger than those that extend our joints outwards, and
therefore we are for ever trying to go back to the position we
were in before we were born. The hands are no exception
and if you look at any six people I will guarantee most of
them will be sitting with their legs crossed and their hands
folded together.

The worst thing you can do is what so many static older
people do; hold a tissue in your hands and sit squeezing it. I
beg of you, sit with your hands open and if you want to do
something with them, from time to time, open them out *more*
and lift the tips up off whatever they are resting on.

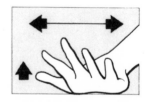

People usually say 'oh yes, I keep my hands moving'. But
the point is they are moving inwards in the *wrong direction* –
making more deformity, and annoying the joints by these

continuous, small ineffectual movements. They should be doing large, easy, full movements in *all directions* very slowly and thoroughly; then the hands can have a complete rest in the extended position. Your reward will be more useful hands, because you will find they come together quite easily when you want them to work. You might try lifting up the fat on the front of your thighs as you lie in bed. You will strengthen your hands and loosen the nasty fat.

Apart from exercises, please find some work for your hands to do several times a day: washing smalls in warm water, playing draughts or bowls, playing any musical instrument, doing carpentry, fixing an electric plug, anything that requires dexterity. It was for this that your hands were made. See list of books (p. 117) for handicrafts.

Beware of lifting heavy objects in your fingers. These can strain the joints. Heavy mixing bowls can be disastrous – try plastic ones. If you have to lift a heavy casserole clamp the whole of each palm on either side of it using oven gloves. Don't just use fingers and thumbs.

If you examine the bones of the fingers you will see they simply lie end to end and therefore can be dislodged by pressure. If this happens and you really stretch the rather fine ligaments surrounding them, then they cannot be put back again into alignment.

Be sure you keep your fingers warm. Because they have no muscles in them – only tendons and bones – they don't have a very good blood supply. So, please, warm gloves outside, woollen mittens in the house if necessary, warm rooms, and keep your arms moving. Do you remember, I wonder, how the old cabbies of the horse-drawn cabs used to sit up on the box exposed to all weathers? They used to flap their arms about, heaved them out and then flung them across their chest, time and time again. They were keeping their hands warm, otherwise they couldn't feel the reins to drive the horse. Take a tip from them. Do the same movement.

Some people who have stiff hands insult them by grasping the stiff joint with the other hand and trying to waggle it about. They even let other people push and exert pressure on the suffering joints. *Never force finger joints.* Try this experiment and you will see why. Open out your hand with the palm facing you. Now bend each finger in turn quickly, and see where it touches your palm if you just let it go where it wants.

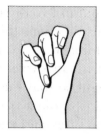

You will be surprised to find they all touch exactly the same spot – just at the root of the thumb. Why? Because every joint of every finger, which means twelve joints in all, is arranged at a slightly different angle so as to bring the finger tips across the palm for holding objects. You will never, therefore, be able to manipulate each joint along its correct axis because you do not know the exact direction in which each moves, although each moves like a hinge. You are in great danger of destroying the joint by pushing it out of its true alignment, especially if it already has any degree of deformity. *Beware, keep off.*

Your Wonderful Thumb

Shake out your hand loosely and then let it lie in front of you, palm uppermost. You will find the thumb is resting in the line of your first finger on the top of your palm. You are the only animal whose thumb lies like that – the apes all have their thumb lying *beside* the first finger, not on top of it. Only the human thumb can touch the tip of the first finger. Our thumbs are able to work much more intimately with the fingers, and achieve complicated activities such as turning a key. You may find it difficult to believe, but it is a fact that the area in the brain to send orders to and receive feelings from the thumb is larger than that for the whole trunk (see p. 32, *Simple Movement*).

The joint of the thumb nearest the wrist is saddle shaped. This means it is scooped out in two directions and is therefore very free-moving. The directions this joint can move in are: (1) towards your first finger, (2) straight forward away from that finger, and (3) it can swivel towards your little finger keeping quite straight so that the two pads 'oppose' each other. Using its final two joints as well the thumb can also bend up into the palm or extend and open out beyond the hand. The thumb is therefore a most versatile member, capable of the most intricate work, which I hope you encourage it to perform.

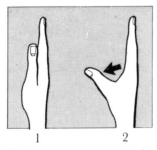 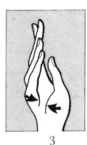

To do all these movements the thumb has muscles controlling it lying in the lower arm, which, after becoming tendons, pass over the wrist. To assist these there are also small muscles which make the bulge where your thumb meets the wrist. On the other side of your hand there is a lesser bulge where there are a few muscles to move the little finger. If you bring the thumb and little finger towards each other, keeping them straight, you will notice how the hollow of the palm is deepened.

From this description you can work out all the special movements to do to strengthen the thumb muscles, and preserve its joints so that they can move easily.

Thumb Movements

Begin with the back of the hand on a table, then:

1 Press hard against first finger keeping thumb straight. Remind yourself this is a sign of the unique human hand. Use it.

2 Lift straight up towards your nose. Because the thumb naturally lies on the first finger, this lifting movement is the one most easily lost. Persevere with it.

3 Take across palm so that the little finger and thumb pads approach together. Keep finger and thumb straight. Another human movement: cherish it.

4 Bend down across palm. You may like to make a little circle with the top of the thumb across the palm. You are flexing your three thumb joints.

5 Extend and open far from fingers. You may like to extend and open out all the fingers at the same time.

Remember, the working hand must not be helped. It works on its own. Rest whenever you like. If you find the movements difficult, try doing them in a basin of warm water. Be very careful of that saddle joint of the thumb nearest to the wrist. Because it is so mobile, and used so much, this joint is the one which most often becomes deformed. Make good use of your hands; they enjoy being used, and should give you enjoyment. They hate to lie crushed on your lap, still and useless, gradually becoming incapable of any feeling except pain.

Mirror Following

You may enjoy playing this game which will encourage you to experience the sensitivity of your hands and at the same time increase muscle activity of your hands and arms in a pleasant, amusing way. You sit opposite a partner who performs movements of the hands and arms while you follow, as in a mirror. Vary slow with quick movements. Then change over. It's more entertaining if done to music.

5

TAKE CARE OF YOUR

Hips, Legs, Posture and Balance

Legs are for standing on, for transferring your weight to the ground as you sway about, and for propelling your weight in any direction you wish. We will, therefore, find heavier muscles all the way down them and we will ask them to do heavier exercise. Are your legs strong enough to do all this easily?

Every step we take, we put our full weight on one leg as the other leg lifts forward. All sports and dancing mean swaying from one leg to the other, and very few people stand evenly on both legs – usually they bend one very slightly and put all the weight through the other. So we are going to have to maintain very hefty muscles around the hip and knee to do all this work. If we are wise, we will watch our weight, and try to stand with our weight evenly on both legs, not over-burdening our leg joints.

The easiest way to strengthen these muscles is by swimming, or in bed or in the bath where the weight of the leg is being supported. The strongest way is to work them against the weight of your whole body, as in heel raising, knee bending (p. 67). Between these two extremes you can move each leg by itself, so that it just carries its own weight, though you can later add to this by wearing a heavy shoe and then increasing the load by bandaging a weight to the shoe. Choose for yourself what you find suitable and progress from that.

THE HIP

Your hip joint is the most stable joint of your whole body. The top end of the big leg bone (femur) is shaped like a ball. It fits snugly into a socket in the pelvis, and therefore can be moved in all directions. It has very strong ligaments both inside and outside the joint, and so it is practically impossible to dislocate it, in contrast to your versatile and easily dislocated shoulder joint. The latter is for movement, the former for power.

Hip Movements

Standing holding onto a strong support:

1 Bend your leg up towards your nose with the knee bent.

2 Extend the leg far back, keeping your trunk upright.

3 Push the leg out to the side. Keep the foot facing forward. You use these muscles when you stand on one leg.

4 Keeping its heel fixed on the ground, swivel your leg outwards and inwards, keeping it straight.

If you find simple movements boring to do, then add music – you can always get some rhythm from the radio. I hope you progress to dancing in any form you enjoy, or tennis, indoor or outdoor bowls, gardening or walking the dog, increasing to hilly walks and stair climbing as you feel able. By the way, walking downhill or downstairs is very strong work for your leg muscles.

THE KNEE

Instead of being made like a ball and socket and so capable of movements in all directions, the knee is the point at which the large thigh bone is just balancing on top of the lower leg bone and damage may occur by force being awkwardly directed through it. Damage will always cause swelling around the joint. If you have any swelling you should see your doctor, and should not do any extra exercise till he says so.

The main movements are hingelike, i.e. backwards and forwards. But you can also rotate at the knee. Sit down, bend your knee to a right angle, and put your heel on the floor. Now place your finger tips on the tendons under your knee on either side. Turn your foot inwards and outwards and you will feel the tendons tighten alternately like the reins on a horse as your whole lower leg rotates to each side.

Knee Movements

1 Easiest of all: 'Quadriceps contractions'. Begin sitting with your knee bent or lying straight. Straighten your knee as fully as possible. Then, with your toes tilted towards your face, make a final effort to pull your knee cap further upwards, so that your knee straightens still more.

This is a most useful exercise because it keeps your knee safe when standing, if you are tending to lose balance. If you feel tightness behind the knee when you attempt it, it means you have been keeping your knee bent and everything at the back of the knee has got a bit stiff. *Do not rub it.* There are several large blood vessels near the surface there. Proceed carefully with slow bending and stretching. In time you may be able to get it fully straight. It will then be much more comfortable. Knees easily stiffen because there are so many little bags of fluid and bags of fat tucked under and around the tendons and the joint. To keep these flexible, as they are meant to be, you have to keep the knee active so that the bags (bursae) are alternately squashed and released.

2 Concentrate on bending and stretching your knee as gently but as fully as you can – especially the final straight-

ening with your foot tilted towards your face. It is tempting to give the leg a push with your hand but please resist the idea. Instead think what *movement* you want to achieve, e.g. if you are lying in bed on your side think 'I will bend my lower leg gently so that my foot is aiming to touch my bottom'. Try doing this slowly and thoroughly, then quickly with a swinging motion – bend – stretch – bend – stretch. Also try doing it with both legs at the same time. Place one on top of the other. I have also found this a most satisfactory way of exercising both hips and knees at the same time when they are unable to bear full weight. You direct your knees to move up towards your nose while your feet aim towards your bottom. Follow this by a full stretch of your legs and spine. This is very safe and comforting in a warm bed.

3 When sitting do a few of the rotations (p. 66) with your knee at a right angle and your heel only on the ground. This lubricates the joint nicely in a safe way.

4 For really strong work hold onto a heavy piece of furniture or the kitchen sink, and with your head held tall and your back straight, rise as high as you can onto your toes, then sink slowly, with your knees turned out and your bottom being lowered exactly over your heels. Go just a little way down, then stretch your hips and knees fully. The top of your head should be directed straight up to the ceiling, eyes looking forward. Then lower your heels. This exercise is called Heel-Raising, Knee-Bending. As you get stronger you can sink lower when bending your hips and knees, but don't attempt too much or you may fall over.

You are really practising for lifting anything, be it a milk bottle from the doorstep or the shopping. It is wiser not to attempt to lift grandchildren from the toddler stage onwards; instead sit down and encourage them to climb onto your lap.

When lifting anything, lower yourself down with your

back straight, bending hips and knees, then come up in the same way, back still straight, and holding the object as close to your body as possible. It is dangerous just to bend over with your head leading and your knees stiff, grasping what you want ahead of you. Your heavy head may pull you over, or you may damage your back. Instead, work from your *hips*. Never kneel down on a hard floor or you may damage the knee joints. Kneel on a cushion.

ANKLES AND FEET

This is a very common place for rheumatic pain as, of course, all your weight passes through these joints. Be sure you wear really well-fitting lace-up shoes with thick yet flexible rubber soles if you have this trouble. It is kind to your suffering joints.

The ankle bends your foot up and down, but when it is in the down position, due to the shape of the joint, it will also allow the foot to waggle inwards and outwards. When you bend the foot up and then try the same movement, you will find it moves less freely and that all movement takes place in the foot itself rather than the ankle joint. You should, therefore, carry out all these four movements (up, down, inwards, outwards) gently and thoroughly.

Feet often become very stiff because people give them so little varied lubricating movement, but such a lot of hard work carrying their weight around. Too often, people bump their feet, bang – bang – bang, as they walk and hardly move at the ankles at all. Please walk heel-toe, bending both your ankle and foot on every step; otherwise, it is as though you were hitting your foot with a ten-stone hammer (i.e. your weight) each time you put your foot down and land your weight onto it. Treat feet gently and with respect.

Your foot, like your hand, has a selection of little bones in front of the ankle joint – seven, in fact – all ready with mobile joints for you to put your weight gradually through if you will just keep them well oiled with proper movement. Then further forward are the five bones, as in the hand, leading to the toes. The arrangement of the muscles controlling the toes is very similar to that in the hand.

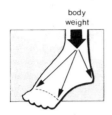

body weight

When your weight hits your foot, one half of it goes straight through your heel into the ground, one quarter goes along the line of your big toe and the other quarter spreads out forward over the other four toes. So you see – you stand on a kind of tripod with the weight evenly distributed. Do you do that? Or do you just bump along as though your foot were a piece of wood? Later, I will detail all the movements you should do to keep your feet strong and mobile.

If the tendons from your leg muscles controlling your toes, and the small muscles of your feet are not doing their job of holding up the arches of your feet, the arches *spread* and you have pain. Your toes then tend to knock against the lining of your shoes and a bunion or a hammer toe can develop very easily. Also hard skin toughens to protect your foot from the pressure. If you already have a bunion or hammer toe, get some animal wool from the chemist. This is raw wool from sheepskin. Tease it out into strands, and twist these around the protruding bony parts of your foot. This will give you great relief, as it makes a very squashy covering. Never use ordinary cotton wool. It balls with the perspiration from your feet and causes further damage. As you wash your feet daily in warm water – no soaking please – also wash out the animal wool and use it again when dry. Examine your feet for any cuts or swelling or darkened colour. Always cover any abrasion with a Bandaid and if swelling or change of colour persists, take it to your doctor.

Do always dry your feet very carefully and rub in some cream or cocoa nut oil if the skin is dry or dab with surgical spirit if sweaty and damp, especially between the toes. Use a fine pumice stone on hard skin to get rid of it. Corn plasters can be dangerous. If you have definite corns you must see a chiropodist and also examine your shoes for faulty pressure. But prevention is better than cure, so choose shoes that do not squash your toes together and develop the strength of the small muscles of your feet as well as the pulling power of the tendons crossing the bones under your feet. In this way you will have healthy mobile *arched* feet. These arches distribute your weight evenly through your foot without damage, as they are arranged from back to front and from side to side. Here is how to preserve them. In your bath or in bed or at any time when you are in a warm carpeted room, remove your shoes and stockings and do the following:–

Movements of Ankles, Feet and Toes

1 Curl in your toes and bend your foot down and inwards. Waggle it from side to side.

2 Extend and open out your toes and bend up your foot. Waggle it from side to side. Shake your foot if you feel it is going to cramp and begin again.

3 Circle your foot, bending your toes when your foot is down and opening and extending them when your foot points upwards. Circle in each direction, making as wide a circle as you can with your big toe. Shake your foot to rest it.

4 Place your foot on the ground, bed, end of bath, wher-

ever you happen to be and, keeping your heel down, curl in your toes, humping up the middle of your foot as high as you can. Lay the toes out flat, stretching them as much as possible. Repeat as often as you wish, but don't overtire the tiny muscles as you train them.

5 Now keep your toes out quite straight and hump up the knuckles of your toes so that you shorten your foot. Do this slowly and thoroughly and then quickly and easily. You can then do it at any time *inside your shoes* when standing at the sink or at a bus stop. All this also helps the circulation of blood from your feet back to your heart. When you lie down for a rest, have your feet just about twelve inches higher than your hips.

Of course you are already attending to the skin of your feet (p. 16). You have nice square-cut nails, and shoes that support your feet and yet bend on each step.

Foot exercise and care are not an end in themselves. They are just preparation so your legs and feet can comfortably move you about any way you want; so be sure they take you out for a walk *every day*.

SITTING DOWN AND STANDING UP

It is amazing how many people fall when trying to sit down. They approach the chair, turn their back to it, aim their bottom at it, miss, and down they go. Instead, walk straight up to the chair until the front of your legs are touching it. Then park your stick(s) or crutch(es) on the back of the chair, if using them, hold the arms as you turn around and, *keeping your head high*, slowly sit well back into the chair so that your hips and knees take your weight as much as possible and your arms also help to lower you.

When you want to stand up, slide to the front of the chair,

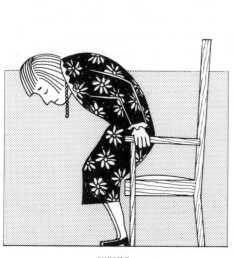
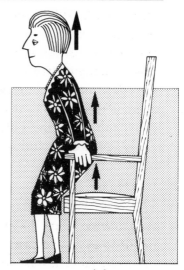

wrong   *right*

one buttock after the other, grasp the chair arms, hold your head *up*, and, with your feet near the chair and one slightly in front of the other, push on your arms. As you rise with a straight back, strongly straighten your hips. Remember they are the strongest muscles in your body. Use them to lift yourself.

Too many people hang their heavy heads down, with their spine curled forward and attempt to heave themselves upwards with bent hips and knees. This is dangerous and can easily lead to a fall. Practise standing and sitting often, gradually putting less weight on your arms and more on the legs.

Getting In and Out of a Car

People often find it difficult to get in or out of a car, and can easily wrench a knee if they are not careful. The car should be parked about one foot away from the pavement to allow one to step to and from the gutter. This gives you valuable extra depth. When the door has been opened, stand facing outwards with the back of your legs touching the side of the seat. Do not attempt to twist on your legs into the car but sit down facing outwards. Then lift your knees and swivel on your bottom to face forwards. Put your feet down and you are safely in. You get out by the same method in reverse order, also into the gutter.

For getting in and out of bed, see p. 98.

POSTURE

A healthy old age means preserving, as much as possible, our normal good habits of activity that we had in our youth. So many facilities are lost by people who say, 'Oh, it's just my age', when it is nothing of the kind. It is often simply because they have stopped using their body naturally. It certainly isn't natural to slump in a padded chair for hours on end, and it plays havoc with our posture and balance.

When we talk about Good Posture and Bad Posture, what do we mean? Good posture means that, when standing, you are conveying your weight through to your feet with as little strain as possible anywhere on your body, and all your weight is evenly balanced. Each part of your body should be in the best position for it to function well. Your head should be held high and straight so the brain gets a good blood supply and your sight and hearing are not impaired. Your chest and abdomen should not be squashed, so have your spine stretched and your chest lifted.

A good sitting posture means you are using the pelvic bones and as much of your thigh bones as possible to receive your weight evenly. This depends on the size of the seat. Your chest and abdomen should be free to do their work without being cramped, and preferably your head and arms should be supported.

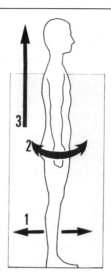

Here is how to obtain a good standing posture. (1) Stand and sway gently forward and back at your ankles until you feel your weight moving. Then let the weight pass down through the middle of your feet just in front of your ankles. Let your knees sag very slightly; do not brace them back. (2) Adjust your pelvis so that it is neither dropped too far down in front, nor too far up – just gently poised in the middle. (3) Now stretch right up your back to the top of your head, keeping your eyes looking straight forward and your chin at a right-angle to your neck. Your ears should be directly above your shoulders and your arms hanging quite loosely.

Now, try walking: put your heels down first; move freely from your hips, your head held high and your arms gently swinging, opposite hand and foot. You may feel rather silly at first, but you will look marvellous, and all your spinal joints, your chest and your internal organs will be free to function properly instead of being pressed upon and cramped. Try to walk outside like this every day, in all weathers. Just dress to suit the weather. Older people may feel they are getting shorter; this is often because they slump instead of stretching, and they have allowed their back, neck and tummy muscles to get weak. Also, they may suffer from chronic fatigue through inactivity and poor breathing, possibly also meagre diet.

BALANCE

It is vital to preserve your balance: the ability to sway your weight but to be able to control it so you don't fall over. This is essential for healthy, safe living. Many people die or break bones every year from falls in their own homes, so keep on doing all exercises and daily movements that will keep you safe when swaying. But be careful as you practise.

Control of balance may be grossly interfered with by any operation which involves much cutting of the nerves conveying sensation from joints and muscles to the spine and lower brain. This may be an abdominal, spinal or leg operation. During recovery, a new pattern of receiving messages from that area to the brain has to be established. This can usually be achieved by practice, perseverance and time.

Continuous pain over a long period may easily cause faulty posture. One shifts the body weight as it is being transferred to the feet, so that pressure on the painful area is minimised. Try to avoid doing this any more than is absolutely necessary, or you may cause further trouble to yourself. When the pain has been cured or controlled, examine your posture frequently in a long mirror and be sure you correct it completely for your future comfort. Here is a safe exercise to strengthen back and legs.

Five Holes in the Bed

This exercise is marvellous for strengthening the muscles of the back, especially if you have sometimes to rest in bed because of some mechanical reason.

Lie flat without any pillows or as few as possible. You are going to aim to make five dents in the mattress by pressing into its resistance with your head, heels, elbows or hands. You can begin pushing into the bed at any one of these, then hold this position, pushing continuously while you add the others.

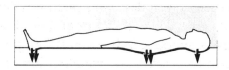

It is surprisingly hard work and you will tend either to arch up your spine, or hold your breath, or both. Do not do either. If you hold your breath, you put up the pressure in your abdomen – instead, sing or count. If you arch, you only get movement in your spine and what you are aiming at is *power* in your back muscles. This is why you are working against the resistance of the mattress. This exercise is most successful on any kind of mattress, and helps you stand up straight when you get up.

The Plantar Reflex

We have many normal reflexes to help us maintain our upright balance. A reflex is a response by muscle work to a nerve stimulation of some kind. Blinking your eye when something is going into it, is a good example. Your eye sees the object but before the information has reached your conscious brain, the muscles have got the message via the local nerves and worked to close the eye. Reflexes always work if they are repeated.

The reflex that is going to help you with your posture and balance is the Plantar Reflex: pressure on the soles of the feet causes the extensors of the legs and the back muscles to work strongly. You have probably experienced it when you have held a baby in your arms. If he pressed his feet on your hand he would immediately stretch backwards. This automatic movement happens so quickly that it can be quite frightening. Lying for a long time in bed is very bad for your posture because you cease to stimulate your plantar reflex. So get up often and walk in bare feet. Wear proper shoes, not soft bedroom slippers, indoors. When you stand, press your feet down and assist your reflex by straightening and lengthening your back.

Another reflex which controls balance is the Stretch Reflex: when a muscle is stretched it responds by working and shortening itself. If you are beginning to fall to one side, the muscles at the other side begin to be stretched; they immediately contract and shorten to bring you upright again.

Try now. Stand on one leg and hold onto a strong piece of furniture. Sway about, pressing your supporting foot down firmly. When you feel safe, take your hand off the support, go on swaying. Then try on the other leg. Later raise your arm and look around as you sway.

The ability to balance and also to recover your balance when it begins to waver will save you, one day, from a dangerous fall. You should be able to wobble safely at all times.

Keep standing up to wash and dress, especially to put on socks or stockings or pants. If necessary dress beside your bed so if you think you are losing your balance, with one leg off the ground, you can quickly fall onto the bed (p. 44). But if you preserve your power to sway safely you should be able to remain upright. Remember: 'what you don't use, you lose'.

I hope you are playing some sport that requires balance, such as bowls, or dancing of some kind. These are ideal for preserving health, good posture, quickness of body response, body awareness and enjoyment. Movement is the natural response of a healthy body. Try to keep your pace going. You don't need to be slow because you are sixty. Beware of developing the habit of sitting fixed before the television. Pick out ahead some programmes that really interest you, and watch these only. Sit in a good posture as you watch, with your head supported and try not to eat or drink. When your chosen programme is over *switch off*. Get up and go and do something active.

Osteo-Arthritis of Hips and Knees

This common complaint may affect any or all four joints. Often it is one-sided which may possibly be due to our habit of putting all our weight through one leg.

The real cause of osteo-arthritis is unknown, indeed there are many types of it, but so much can be done both to relieve pain and to repair the affected part that medical advice should be sought. Your job is to keep as much weight off the affected part as may be necessary by rest, or using stick or crutches, and yet to preserve as much painless movement there as possible, and keep all the surrounding muscles in working order. Perform the movements suggested here daily beginning with the easiest you can manage and then progressing to stronger if you are able. Stop at once if you have any pain and then try again gently. Of course you do not allow yourself to gain weight. Try to preserve your balance and upright stance when standing, sitting and walking with weight evenly on both legs. Choose soft seats with supporting backs and arms.

Warmth is of the greatest comfort to damaged joints, so

try to have a warm bath daily if you can. An electric blanket is very soothing or a heated pad or a hot water bottle, but be sure to have several layers of wool between you and the heat, so that it is diffused all over the part. Never go to sleep with an electric pad turned on.

Sticks and Crutches

If you have been given sticks or crutches by the physiotherapists in hospital, they will have chosen the right height for you and shown you how to use them. But people often borrow a stick from a friend, or buy one if they feel unsafe. This is not wise as you may weaken your legs even more by its use. You may damage your shoulder or spinal joints and, if you walk badly, you may damage your balance reflexes and lose the ability to walk like a human being. You are then another candidate for a dangerous fall.

The height of the stick or handle of the crutch should be measured from your hand to the ground with the elbow at an angle of about 135 degrees. If they are too short, you strain your spine bending forward and, if too long, you strain your shoulder joints. There should always be a rubber ferrule on the end of sticks.

You should place the stick or crutches *beside* your legs, never in front. If you are using one stick it must be in the hand opposite the affected leg and move exactly when the opposite leg moves. If you allow the stick in front, you are walking as though you have three legs. If you are using two sticks or crutches and allow them in front, you are walking as though you have four legs, like a horse. Either way, you completely lose your normal human walking pattern. Then you really are in danger of falling over.

You should press *down* on the stick or crutches, stretch your back up, hold your head high and walk with a normal

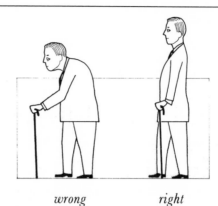

wrong   *right*

gait. Try to put more weight through your legs and less onto the support, when possible. Try to do without the support at home and walk as quickly as possible there, to preserve your agility.

6

TAKE CARE OF YOUR

Breathing, Heart, Belly and Back

Now good digestion wait on appetite and health on both.
SHAKESPEARE, *Macbeth*

It is in the trunk that all the work is done to supply fresh oxygen and food for the whole body and to get rid of its waste. What can we do to make our own supply and rubbish departments more efficient?

The trunk is divided into two very uneven compartments. The chest has about one third of the area and the abdomen two thirds. Between these, there is a large sheet of muscle called the diaphragm, shaped like a mushroom directed upwards, forming the floor of the chest and, therefore, the ceiling of the abdomen. The stalk is attached to the spinal column of bones about the level of your waist. The edges attach to the six lower ribs. The upper surface bulges up to about your fifth ribs, with your lungs on either side and your heart to the left of centre, actually resting on it. Under the diaphragm, inside the ribs and below are the abdominal contents. The liver, a huge, busy organ, lies entirely under the ribs.

THE CHEST

The chest acts like bellows. To be able to do this, it has to change shape and, therefore, it has to have muscles, bones and joints. The twelve pairs of ribs enclose and protect the heart and lungs and join at the back on either side onto the twelve bones of the upper back, i.e. the spinal column. In front, the ribs have softish cartilage joining them onto the breast bone which, in turn, is held in place above by the two collar bones attached to it, one on either side, and so it all moves very easily.

If you put your hands gently onto the sides of your rib cage, you will feel it rising and falling. This it does about twelve to twenty times every minute. To make you breathe in, your mushroom-shaped diaphragm slightly flattens its curve downwards and then helps the muscles between your ribs to lift them up and outwards.

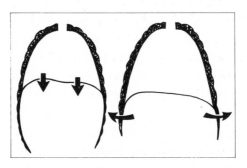

Diaphragm action causing inward breath

Your chest is therefore made bigger downwards, out-wards and upwards, and, because 'nature abhors a vacuum', the outside air, laden with oxygen, rushes in. The lungs are composed of tiny air passages and millions of tiny blood vessels. The change over of oxygen into the blood, and waste carbon dioxide out of it takes place between these myriad tiny blood vessels and the air in the passages. When the muscles stop working and relax, the ribs fall back against the lungs, the diaphragm rises upwards and presses on them from below and so the air is squeezed out.

Breathing is so important that you have several breathing centres in your subconscious lower brain monitoring it at any moment without you having to control it consciously. You have slow breathing during sleep, quick breathing for activity and special kinds for sneezing, coughing, laughing etc. But you can also control the breathing muscles yourself if you wish. Very few people breathe as thoroughly as they should, so you ought to do this every day. Here is how to get the best and most efficient breathing.

Sit down, and rest your head backwards, place your hands gently on either side of your lower chest, so that your finger tips just gently touch each other in front, above your waist. Now breathe in consciously, expanding your lower chest outwards, and you will feel the upper part of your abdomen, under your finger tips, bulge forwards slightly from the increase of pressure caused by the descent of the diaphragm. You can also encourage and feel the ribs lift sideways and upwards towards your armpits. Then stop, breathe out easily and feel the ribs fall down and inwards and the tummy fall backwards.

Do this twice or at most three times. If you do it too often you may upset your breathing centres and feel giddy. You can repeat it later. The reason you put your hands on the middle and lowest part of your chest is because there is the widest part of your rib cage and you get most movement of the ribs there. Of course, the air goes into the whole area of the lungs just as it does into a balloon when you blow it up. The walls of all the little passages in your two lungs would cover a tennis court if they were spread out. This is about forty times the surface area of the skin of your whole body. Why is there this massive arrangement for exchange of carbon dioxide for oxygen into the blood? Because every single cell of your body needs it to stay alive and working.

Please sit and think about these amazing facts and then I

am sure you will not find doing deep breathing every day a waste of time. You will also appreciate why smoking is such a bad idea.

THE HEART

The heart is a pump. Exercise of any kind makes your heart stronger because more blood is sent back to the heart in the veins as the exercise proceeds, and so the heart has to pump more strongly to push it up into the lungs and after it has been aerated there, into the aorta, the huge artery leading from the heart which, eventually, via its branches, takes blood all over the body. Using the larger groups of muscles strongly forces this process greatly. This is called aerobic exercise, and should be sustained for lengthening periods of time, during training.

It has been found however that gentle exercise, performed for short bouts about three times a week, helps the heart to develop strength. Like any other muscle, it grows strong by being used; otherwise, it becomes flabby and is apt to get fat around it. It is only necessary for people over fifty years to use 50 per cent of their capability to get maximum benefit. Over-exercise is unnecessary.

Ask your doctor if you are fit to take some easy exercise, such as walking, stair-climbing and arm and leg movements. This can then lead to your favourite sport or dancing. If you are in normal health, I am sure he/she will be glad to agree.

Experts tell us we should make ourselves slightly breathless by some kind of exercise every day – just enough so that we can feel our breathing speeding up but yet are still able to talk. Try it – even if you have to be in bed for any mechanical reason (osteo-arthritis of the spine or hip, for instance). You can swing your arms up and down and around or, if you have to sit a lot, then twist and turn your body and don't forget deep breathing for everyone. Little and often is the best recipe to reverse weakness into general well-being. As you feel better – and you will – increase what you do.

THE BACK AND TUMMY MUSCLES

We have already spoken (p. 24) about the seven bones in your neck supporting your head and now we must look at the bones below that. There are twelve in your upper back, five in your lower back, and then your pelvis below. This is your spine (vertebral column). It has a hollow centre containing the spinal cord. This is composed of the nerves from all over your body going to and from your brain.

The bones are piled on each other rather like cotton reels, getting bigger the lower they go as they accumulate the weight of your body. As well as the moveable joints, between each bone is a pad of gristle called a disc – you may have heard of one slipping! They are attached above and below to the bones and if used frequently are squashed as the bones move and then recover their shape again. This keeps them mobile.

Usually the 'slipped disc' is caused by someone doing a sudden movement he or she is not accustomed to do and the disc is caught between the bones instead of returning smoothly into place. You can get this at any age. The safe thing to do is to move your spine gently and fully every day so that the joints are accustomed to movement and the muscles which move them are strong and elastic.

Some of these muscles are the ones we call the tummy muscles – those in front of the abdomen. If you remember they always have a layer of fat in front of them and another layer behind them, I don't think you will need much encouragement from me to do the movements. You will certainly make your front flatter and stronger, as well as making your

spine safer for other activities. It should also help you get rid
of flatulence and constipation. These are often found in
people who spend a lot of time lying, or sitting curled into a
bundle in a padded armchair.

Stretching

(A) is how your spinal column should be shaped. But with
your heavy head on top pressing down, your heavy arms
heaving forward, and possibly with some thinning of your
bones (p. 18), plus flabby muscles and disinterest, you are
apt to look like (B) as/you get older. But there is no need. As
you can see, what these joints need most of all is *stretching*.

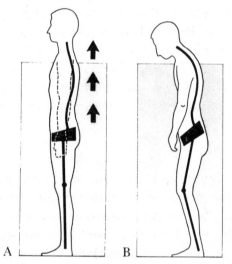

Whether you are in bed, sitting or standing, stretch –
stretch – stretch, the top of your head going up towards the
ceiling. Keep your eyes facing forward and you may be
amazed to find you are looking at a point quite two inches
above what you were before. Rest – then stretch again and,
this time, complete the movement of the Three-Point Pull.

As you stretch your head *up*, pull your two shoulders *down* (see p. 25). This gives you a beautiful long neck with your head poised above it.

Now, to strengthen muscles. The muscles of your back lie closely on either side of the column. Some reach your head and some go out round your chest on either side; one even reaches your arm bone and pulls it back. So, let's use them all. Begin doing the movements below, sitting upright in a chair or in bed. Later, try to do them standing as your balance improves.

THE BACKWARDS STRETCH

Pull your head, chest and arms backwards, making your spine curve gently backwards. Now stretch upwards again and have a rest. Repeat if you want to. I usually find I enjoy the second or third movement better than the first. If lying in bed, do the 'Five holes in the bed' (p. 26) as well.

All the other movements are going to be especially for your tummy muscles. The back muscles join in when they can.

THE CURL

Tuck your chin in and curl your head and spine forwards. Breathe out strongly and you will feel your tummy tightened as you do so. Now uncurl, breath in and stretch up. Repeat as you wish. You have now used all your spinal joints in backwards and forwards directions.

We will use next all the joints that move you in other directions. This will really bring into play all your tummy muscles very thoroughly. The sheet of muscle over your abdomen is attached to your spine at the back, ribs above, and pelvis below. Its various strands are formed like a Union Flag. To make it neat, and tight which we all want, and help it to support your back, we have to shorten each stripe:

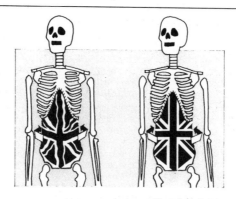

*Result of
shortening exercises*

THE TWIST

Put your arms across your chest. This is where the twisting takes place. Twist around so that instead of facing the wall in front you face the side wall. Breathe out strongly. Stretch your body upwards and breathe in. Spin around to face the opposite wall breathing out. Repeat as you wish to both sides.

THE SIDE BEND

Put your hands on your waist where the movement is going to take place and bend sideways. Breathe out. Stretch up while breathing in. Repeat to the other side, and as often as you wish again to either side, up to a limit of one or two minutes, no more. But you must do all the movements and the breathing.

Warning: never do double leg raising and lowering or bicycling in the air. It is a most dangerous exercise partly because it raises the abdominal pressure so much and can cause hernia, back damage, and pelvic damage in women resulting in strain on the supporting structures of the womb. (For a full explanation see *Simple Movement* by Laura Mitchell and Barbara Dale, pp. 61–65.)

INSIDE THE ABDOMEN

Now let us take a look inside the abdomen. There is so much there that it is like an overfull suitcase. The consequent pressure keeps everything in its place but has some disadvantages. One of these can be incontinence of faeces or urine or both.

Incontinence

Incontinence of urine is unfortunately a fairly common complaint in the over fifties. It means that you cannot control the bladder exit and urine leaks from it either continuously or on any sudden increase of pressure in the abdomen. This can be brought on by laughing or coughing, etc. The cause may simply be the general weakening of muscle which tends to happen in inactive over fifties. This condition can always be helped and often cured. People who are slow in walking for any reason, often have difficulty in reaching the lavatory in time. They also should read on.

There are exercises you can do to strengthen the muscles surrounding the bladder and the little canal leading to the outside exit. They are very simple and suitable for both men and women. If you are having this most uncomfortable trouble do try these first. If they don't help you, see your doctor, who can put you in touch with experts in the Disabled Living Foundation in London. There are now Incontinence Specialists being trained all over the country. The following exercises are suitable to control incontinence of urine or faeces.

1 When you are passing urine try to stop and start the stream several times.

2 When sitting or lying try to tense and pull in your anus (the exit from the bowel) as though you were trying to stop

passing a motion. Do not use your buttocks: the muscles are inside your pelvis. Hold tightly for a count of five. Rest then repeat.

3 Do Exercise 2 and add more tensing and pulling up into yourself further forward, so you are lifting and squeezing the whole floor of muscle inside. You will be using the same actions you felt when stopping the stream of urine, as all the loose, floppy fat inside is gathered together, and rises tightly upwards.

Do Exercises 2 and 3 for about one minute and repeat as often as possible all day long – sitting, knitting, watching television, standing at the sink, waiting for a bus, in bed before sleep etc. It may take you about a month to feel the difference but it is worth persevering.

If you are too fat for your height this can also be a cause of incontinence. It puts up the pressure inside your abdomen. So do consider reducing your weight by eating less of everything, especially fat. You might like to try the popular fibre diet. See page 87 for tummy muscle exercises.

Eating (or Diet)

Now we come to supply and waste departments. That means your entire food canal – mouth, stomach, small and large bowels; and also liver, etc. The food you eat is gradually churned into a fluid that can be absorbed into the blood stream through the walls of the small intestine (bowel). The food then goes via the blood to the liver where it undergoes further processes and finally from there, it continues all over the body dissolved in the blood, so that millions of cells of all different kinds of which you are made, may be nourished and regrow to keep you healthy. Yesterday's cheese and potatoes become quite literally part of your own body cells today.

So what does your body require to maintain itself and to give it warmth and energy? Does it matter what you eat? It certainly does. Tea and biscuits, which some older people get into the habit of eating as a meal, starve your body. Here is what you need to replace your worn-out cells, give you plenty of energy, and also defend you against infection and other ills. You need a mixture of these every day.

PROTEINS

To repair your body cells, especially if you are recovering from any illness. You find these in meat, chicken, fish, eggs, milk products, bread, rice, lentils, beans, peas, nuts.

FATS

Fats are very concentrated forms of energy food. Therefore you do not need so much of them daily and you can safely eat less of them to reduce weight. You find them in milk and everything made from milk, also bacon, fat meat, eggs, lard, oil, margarine, nuts. I always use low fat margarine, skimmed milk, low fat cheese and low fat live yoghurt and I always grill and never fry. I have also a magic brush 'Salter's Cook Brush' which absorbs fat, and which I use to stir stews and so take out the fat. All these dodges save calories and improve my palate. I now find fat very cloying and that it spoils different tastes.

SUGAR AND STARCH

These are really the same thing except that starch – also called carbohydrates – is more complicated and takes more digesting. You need some form of sugar to provide energy, but it is wiser to choose things like bread (preferably whole-meal) rather than sweets, biscuits or cakes. You get more health for your money in bread and potatoes as they contain protein, vitamins, iron, fibre and calcium as well as the starch. As well as bread and potatoes you get healthy sugar in porridge, cornflakes, Weetabix, peas, beans, honey, home-made jam, turnips, carrots and fruit of all kinds. Choose these if you need to put on weight.

VITAMINS

Vitamin A

Fights infection and helps keep skin and eyes healthy. You get it in margarine, butter, milk, liver, green vegetables, carrots.

Vitamin B Group

There are several of these and they are needed to digest fats and starches to provide energy. They also feed your nerves. You get them in liver, kidneys, bacon, bread, milk, cheese.

Vitamin C

Fights infection and heals wounds. You need some every day because your body cannot store it. You get it in tomatoes, lettuce, grapefruit, oranges, lemons, blackcurrants, blackberries, rose hip syrup, potatoes, green vegetables – steamed not boiled. Just put them in a sieve and hook it over the pan in which your potatoes – scrubbed but not skinned – are boiling. Put a plate on top to keep in the steam and then you have a hot plate ready to eat from.

Vitamin D

This is essential to calcium being laid down in your bones to prevent them becoming brittle (p. 18). You get it from sunlight and sardines, kippers, margarine, cheese.

MINERALS

Small quantities of these – iodine, potassium calcium, phosphorus, iron, sodium etc. are found in many foods which is why you should have a variety every day. You will then get a mixture of these minerals and you will feel much healthier. Ask some of your young friends to tell you how to use herbs for flavouring instead of too much salt. Herbs are now fashionable, easy to buy, and full of minerals.

WATER

Remember you are 60 per cent made of water (see p. 19). Therefore you need to replenish it daily in any form of fluid you prefer: water, soup, tea, coffee, cocoa, a little beer or wine, fruit juices. You cannot absorb any food at all until it has become fluid. You therefore need three to five pints of fluid every day. Yes, *three to five pints*. Remember you also need fluid to form sweat (see p. 16), you lose fluid from your bowels, and each time you breathe out, from your lungs. Your kidneys need fluid to make urine, in which are dissolved the waste products from your blood collected from all over your body.

If you ever have sickness or diarrhoea, for any reason, be sure you drink plenty to replace the lost fluid. Use soup, Bovril or Marmite to replace lost salts. (See Chapter 1.) I always have some made-up vegetable soup in the freezer compartment of the fridge. You can make it any time. All you need is a few varied vegetables, some brown rice, lentils or peas, ten minutes and a sharp knife. Try to have some fresh parsley to make your soup look pretty and supply iron. Add it raw, chopped fine, just before serving.

FIBRE

This is sometimes called roughage. You have to eat daily some substances that you will not actually absorb but which help the mechanics of digestion. (See book list p. 117). Fibre from vegetables, fruit, brown rice, lentils, beans, green salads, potatoes and wholemeal bread form bulk in the large bowel, and help the contents to move on by the waves of contraction, that continually pass along the entire food canal from the mouth to the exit (anus). This prevents constipation and is much safer than expensive aperients which irritate the passage linings. Constipation can also be caused by not going immediately to the lavatory when you feel the urge. The feeling then passes off, and though it may come again later you may not then get a thorough emptying. The best time to develop this habit is in the morning after your first meal. After a night's starvation there is a 'mass movement' along the whole food canal, after the first swallowing of food takes place.

I hope you always cover all food in the fridge or lying out in the kitchen. Of course be sure to wash your hands thoroughly after using the lavatory. Infection from flies and dirty hands is very common and debilitating.

Older people often find it pleasant to have several small meals throughout the day rather than one big one. This is a good idea as it has been found you are less apt to put on weight by doing this. Just be sure you include all the varied, necessary items in your day's diet. Daily exercise also helps to cut down excessive eating.

Always have some essential foods in your store cupboard in case weather or sudden illness make it impossible for you to shop. Tins of fish, meat, milk pudding, soups, packets of cereal, lentils, peas, sultanas, nuts are always useful and keep well.

Good eating is one of the pleasures of life as well as being essential for good health. It can be enjoyed no matter what your age or what the disability that may annoy you. Be sure you indulge in this pleasure by a varied, interesting diet daily, preferably in company, with an attractively set table. Consider joining a cookery class?

7

TAKE CARE IN YOUR

Home

> Oh, to have a little house!
> To own the hearth and stool and all!
> COLUM, 'An Old Woman of the Roads'

As your home is where you spend most time, it is where you should be getting most exercise. There is no need for special clothing or to set aside a special time of day. When you wait for a kettle to boil, hold onto the sink and do heel raising, knee bending (p. 67), or stand on one leg, if you can, and do some arm movements (p. 48). If you are waiting for someone coming for a meal, do a few dance steps, or some deep breathing, or sit and bend and twist your body, if you prefer (p. 88). If you are sitting waiting at the telephone, raise and lower the other arm above your head very quickly or do back extension followed by the forward curl up plus an outward breath (p. 87). Don't just sit there – do something constructive.

Choose what you do yourself as your body feels which part could do with a bit of activity. Body awareness begins at home, and you should be having bouts of deliberate activity throughout the day, inside the house as well as outside.

In the kitchen, try to sit if you have baking to do or many vegetables to prepare and, if you bend forward for some minutes, vary it with a good stretch up of head and arms, plus a back extension (p. 87). You will find this quite exhilarating. I do it often while writing this book.

Choose with care where you keep your bowls, food, and cleaning materials either to save your strength or give you activity, whichever you need. Have lightweight basins and pails to preserve your finger joints, and keep handy those you use often. Don't waste energy looking for things. Keep it for more enjoyable exercise, like a walk in the open air instead of just trudging about your kitchen. You can buy baskets to screw onto the inside of cupboard doors. When you swing open the door, there are the contents in front of you.

Be sure your ironing board and washing-up basin in the sink are the right height for you. When lifting or laying down anything, remember to bend your hips and knees, and keep your back straight, both to go down and to come up (p. 68). Keep the object as close to you as possible. Carry things with a straight arm down by your side, when possible, with your back straight and stretched, and your head held high.

If you have to move any heavy furniture, turn your back on it and, with back straight, push with your bottom and your legs. Use the big, coarse buttock muscles to do the work.

CHAIRS, BEDS AND BATHS

This is a convenient place to consider chairs, beds and baths. Please consider this very carefully because, when you are over sixty, more time is probably spent sitting and lying than walking about, so it matters greatly to your comfort and health. Many chairs are quite unhelpful and too many beds sag. Some people never experience the pleasure of a warm, cleansing bath.

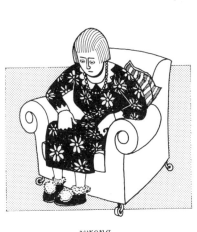
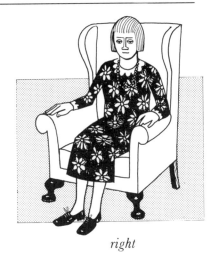

wrong   *right*

Chairs

Chairs should have a deep enough seat for the whole of your leg bones from the knees to the hips to be supported. The chair legs should be the length of your lower legs. It is easy to shorten chair legs by cutting a bit off, or to lengthen them by standing them in wooden cups of suitable length. If you want to be able to move your chair easily, have only two round castors, which move in all directions. Never have castors on all four legs as the chair then moves too easily when you sit down and you may fall.

The back of the chair should be tall enough to support your head and it should also support the curves of your spine. Some people like to put a small pillow behind their waist, but please don't wedge yourself in with too many pillows because I hope you will develop the habit of getting up and moving about every half hour. This is better for your circulation, muscles, joints, digestion, and indeed, morale, than sitting glued to a chair for hours on end. Beware of over-padded chairs which envelop you in a cocoon of inactivity.

Your chair should have arms on which to rest yours. Don't

forget each of your arms weighs as much as your head, i.e. nearly 14 lbs – or a stone of potatoes. When you sit down, you should put all this weight onto the chair and not sit holding it yourself. Sounds silly, doesn't it? But that is what happens when you sit on a chair or settee with no head or arm support.

Beds

The mattress of your bed should support your spine in a straight line when you are lying on your side, and yet support its S curves comfortably when you are lying on your back. We change position about forty times a night and, no matter in what position we lie, the bed should be holding us up. If it sags, we are wasting the energy, as we turn and toss, that sleep is supposed to be restoring in us. I find a foam rubber mattress supports my arthritic spine most comfortably.

If you have disabled legs, you may find the following a helpful way to get onto a bed, instead of sitting on the edge and having someone laboriously lift each leg onto it. I discovered it when I had two painful hips that could not move on their own. Stand beside the bed, fix your hips, then, when you are ready, suddenly sit down, push your body and head strongly backwards and you will find your legs come up onto the bed. You make yourself into a stiff see-saw, so, when your body and especially your heavy head goes down, your legs must come up. You do the trick very quickly so don't let anyone else stand too near or your legs may kick them.

To get out of bed safely and easily, turn onto your side and push yourself upright with your arms, at the same time putting both legs over the edge of the bed. You will then find yourself sitting on the side of the bed. Keep your head upright

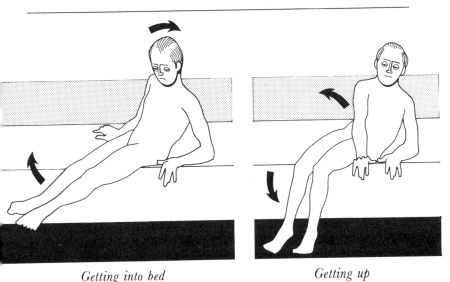

Getting into bed   *Getting up*

all the time. Stay for a few minutes, straightening and bending your knees and ankles until you feel quite in control of yourself. This gives your blood time to get used to running uphill. Then stand with head up and be sure to steady your balance before you walk away, with or without sticks.

Baths

We have already mentioned a wash-down in a basin and washing while on the lavatory (p. 17) but, of course, nothing takes the place of splashing in a nice, warm, deep bath. You may be lucky and have a shower you can use if a bath makes you nervous, or you can attach fitments to your taps for a spray. If these are all impractical, ask your doctor to arrange for the district occupational therapist to call on you and he/she will arrange for a moveable seat, handrail, the essential rubber bath mat and whatever may be necessary, so that you may enjoy the flow of water over your entire body.

This is one of the necessities of healthy living that you must do all you can to continue at any age.

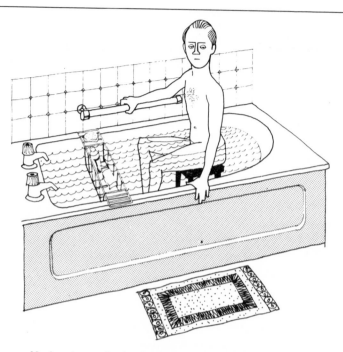

Notice the stool, the depth of water, and the long rail,
supporting the whole of the forearm

GETTING INTO A BATH

If this is difficult, place a towel on the rim of the bath and sit
on it, facing outwards. Then lift the leg nearest to the taps
into the bath, followed by the other, helping with your
hands, if necessary. You will find your bottom easily swings
round on the towel as your legs move. You now place one
hand on each side of the bath, or on the wall rail, if you have
one, and lower yourself down, either onto the little seat in the
bath or forward onto your knees if you are going to lie down
in the water. Then move one leg at a time forward and you
will find yourself lying facing the taps. When you have
washed yourself thoroughly all over with a mild soap and
splashed the warm water all over you generously to your

content, you reverse the above moves to come out again.

Be sure you feel safe on each move before you attempt the next; of course, always have someone else within call, and never lock the bathroom door if you are at all unsure of your movements or balance.

Bedrooms

Your bedroom should have the window open wide to air it every morning and all the bed-clothes taken off and draped over a chair so they may be aired, too, for some hours. If you use a duvet or quilt, shake it out every day and hang it out of the window often to puff up the filling with fresh air.

Some people have the old-fashioned idea that they must sleep with the windows open. If you have any chest condition and, indeed, for most people, this is a bad idea as you simply lie in a cold draught, which no chest enjoys. If you air the bedroom thoroughly during the day, you will have quite enough fresh air to last you through the night, when, in any case, your breathing will be shallow.

SAFETY

Every year, there are more fatal accidents at home than on the roads. Have you carefully considered the safety of your own home? Here are some suggestions:

- Pour boiling water away from you when making tea or filling a hot-water bottle. Lay the bottle on a flat surface and squeeze out the air before putting in the water. This stops it spluttering.
- When carrying a casserole or roast pan, concentrate on what you are doing. Never have a child or animal around your feet at the time. Grasp the dish firmly with your whole

hands – not just fingers – with a really thick cloth between your hands and the heat.

● Frying is a dangerous business, but then I hope you will give it up (p. 91). If you do continue to fry, never, never leave the pan unattended; if you are called away, turn off the heat. Always have one of those fire blankets hanging near the stove.

● First-aid for burns: put your hands at once into cold water. For feet, wring loosely a clean towel in cold water and drape it dripping over the area just as it is. Do not attempt to remove stockings but slip off the shoe, if possible. If a burn is severe, get help and treat for shock.

● Keep your sharp knives high up and have some Band-aid in a handy drawer for a cut you may get suddenly.

● Have a small magnifying glass handy for reading labels, and keep cleaning materials in their own bottles and packets with labels visible and in a safe cupboard.

● Always wipe up any spills on the kitchen or bathroom floor immediately, especially if you use sticks. Talcum powder is particularly slippery.

● Safe, handy rails at the right height can easily be attached to the wall by bath and lavatory. These should be long enough to give support from hand to elbow (p. 100). It is dangerous to cling to towel rails or door handles which often collapse.

● Never have any loose rugs on the floor in the bathroom or elsewhere. Worn areas of carpet are also likely to cause you to trip and fall over. All polished floors are really dangerous. Mirrors should not be placed above fireplaces because of the danger of clothing catching fire. All grates and electric fires should have fireguards. Have large glass ashtrays for any of your visitors who smoke.

● There should be no trailing wires on the floor or worn-out connections with shaky wall plugs. Be sure you take the television plug out of its socket at night. Dark passages or staircases are really dangerous. Get a safe light that can be left on all night. If all your plugs are on the skirting board, consider having any you use often raised higher up the wall. People topple over pulling out a stiff plug from a low socket.

● Please never use folding steps if you are alone in the house. You need someone to steady both you and them when you are window-cleaning, etc. If you can get someone younger to do the job, so much the better.

● Put out your own ration of medicines for the day in a safe cupboard, so you neither overdose nor underdose yourself. Never keep old medicines; give them back to the chemist to dispose of.

● You should devise some way you can call for help, if needed: a telephone near a chair that you could crawl to, a card in the window, three thumps on the wall or floor, etc.

● Finally, when children come to call, be sure you have no dangerous tools, medicines or other hazards lying about.

HYPOTHERMIA

A difficulty peculiar to old age is the inability to register when your temperature is dropping, and you are rapidly losing heat. This is called Hypothermia and can happen out-of-doors or at home, especially to those who do not move about much. The body temperature sinks dangerously low and may lead to unconsciousness and even death. The mechanism in the lower brain below consciousness, that deals with the heat-control reflex, is not working properly.

In the winter of 1982, a national survey was made of over 1,000 elderly people living at home, and it was found that 10 per cent of them had borderline hypothermia. The person affected doesn't realise what is happening. He or she feels rather dazed, weak and uncomfortable, but not actually cold. This happened to me once in winter, when I was gardening, and it was with difficulty that I got into the house and into bed, where I stayed, feeling very odd indeed, for some hours. I was lucky. Sometimes the affected person becomes too apathetic to do anything.

Always see your surroundings are warm enough; 70°F day and night is ideal. 90 per cent of old people live at a temperature below that level. Move about often and, when you go out, wear several layers of woollen clothing. Again, like your skin, these must be scrupulously clean if they are going to trap layers of air to prevent your own heat escaping; softness and fluffiness help this.

Be sure you have a very warm blanket under you in bed, plus bed socks if you have shivery feet. Several layers on top with a feather quilt, alternatively – a duvet, are the best ways of conserving your own heat. Be sure you are warm when you get into bed.

Have you had all the insulation possible done in your home? Old blankets made into linings to curtains, and cling film attached over windows are cheap and successful ways of keeping out the cold. Of course be sure you still get some fresh air.

Cold surroundings and low body temperature lower the resistance of the body to other diseases, especially infection. Old people, therefore, are at great risk in winter from all kinds of illnesses.

TAKE CARE OF THE CARER

Those who look after older people in their own homes are Very Important People and should be appreciated because they have probably sacrificed much to do so. They are saving beds in geriatric hospitals, and are giving the older people what they long for most, which is to stay at home.

The carer should be sure that he or she gets all the necessary back-up facilities of the social services; that he or she also gets out of the house every day, and has frequent days away. Carers must maintain contacts with friends and neighbours, and should encourage the older person to do as much as possible for themselves and others. This preserves their personal dignity.

There should be a sharing of the situation – not dominance by either of the other. The horror of granny-bashing is not a new phenomenon. Beware. Ask for help if you feel the burden of caring is too much. The carers should remember that the care of their own lifestyles (p. 37) in middle age leads to a happy, healthy old age for them in their turn. Consider contacting the National Association of Carers, 58 New Road, Chatham, Kent for advice and information about other services for carers.

8

TAKE CARE OF YOURSELF

in Illness and After

> How agreeable it is to grow older. All I have to do now is relax, keep
> healthy, and let the creative side of my nature take its course.
>
> NOEL COWARD, *Diaries*

Few people are in perfect health all the time. Therefore, from
time to time, to have some form of disability or health
problem is to be one of the majority. By realising this, all
tendency to self pity is immediately removed. If anyone says,
'Why should this happen to me?' I always feel like replying,
'Why not you? It happens to everyone else.'

We should also realise that modern medicine means team-
work, in which the patient is expected to play an important
part. So, how can you take care of yourself when ill, recovering and getting back to normal?

GOING INTO HOSPITAL

Unless you are rushed into hospital following some accident
or emergency, the apprehension caused by waiting can be
great, and the immediate preparations very worrying. Be
sure you ask any questions you want before you go.

If you live with your family or spouse, you can cheerfully
leave the care of the home to them, but, if you live alone,
make a list during your waiting period of all the things you
must see to before you leave. It is just the same as going on

holiday – stop the papers, turn off gas and electricity, arrange for collection of letters and the care of any animal you have, etc. You will have done all this often before, when you were well; now that you are feeling ill, it isn't so easy, so prepare a list beforehand and ask a neighbour to help you check it the day you leave. Give them a duplicate set of keys and ask them if they will collect your letters and see to anything needed in your home. This stops you worrying unduly when you get into hospital, which is very important. You will be sent a list of what to take with you to hospital, but here are some suggestions you may find useful.

Modern hospitals have air-conditioning and are rather hot so, if you can, take only cotton bedwear, and make arrangements for someone to collect, wash and bring them back to you. A long dressing-gown and bedroom slippers are essential for getting up. Take some body cologne – very refreshing – plus plenty of paper tissues and, of course, for women, your usual skin-feeding creams, because the hot, dry air may irritate if you have a sensitive skin.

Take some paperbacks – the hospital library usually goes round the wards only once a week. You will be able to buy a daily newspaper if you wish in the ward. Take a supply of small 'Thank You' cards with the envelopes already stamped. If they are small you don't need to write much, but try to answer every card or present you receive immediately. It shows appreciation and keeps your brain active. You will want extra stamps and writing paper and 5p or 10p pieces for the phone, which is portable so you can use it from your bed. You will probably find that a trolley selling small necessities comes round once a week.

Determine to keep as active as you can when you are in hospital. Move all parts of you not involved with the illness, as freely as possible and do some deep breathing daily. Put your legs apart under the bedclothes – legs tend to come together and the ankles cross, which weakens your walking muscles. Make a habit of stretching your whole body frequently in bed before you go into hospital then you will carry on when you get there. This will help you, when you get up, to look tall and straight, and not bent and crumpled. To prevent bed-sores lift your heels, elbows, bottom and back off the bed from time to time. When you let them rest again on the sheet, feel that they are in a slightly different position. If you can, give these places a rub with your hand to dry off sweat. Skin can be damaged in a few hours if it is allowed to lie heavily in one place, especially if dampened by sweat. Bed-sores are much more easily prevented than cured.

Do remember you are going into hospital of your own free will, to be looked after by people who are professionally trained to do that. Having been in hospital so often, I am continually impressed by the kindness and competence of the various staffs I have met. But remember also that you can ask anything you want to know, and you will get answers. This knowledge is very reassuring before you are admitted, and will certainly help you to take a vital role as part of the team which is trying to get you better. You can be sure everyone there wants you to recover as soon as possible – don't forget there's a queue waiting for your bed! So you need not be afraid you will be detained a single day longer than necessary.

Sometimes people, quite unconsciously, transfer their resentment of their illness or incapacity to the people looking after them, and develop a grudge which impedes their own recovery. Be on the alert against this.

Another little warning. If you are used to sleeping with someone you may find sleep difficult, at first, without the warmth and presence of the other person. Also the narrow bed and sleeping noises from others in the ward may put you off. But you will find you soon get used to the change, and you will certainly be offered a sleeping pill if you wish it.

Everyone's illness takes a slightly different course, so don't get yourself muddled by comparing yourself with other people. Friends are often very keen to tell you what will happen to you because of what happened to Aunt Mary or Uncle George. Listen, but don't let it influence you. You are unique, you will be different. Just determine to take one day at a time and do your best.

VISITING IN HOSPITAL

The most important thing to establish first is that this is not like any ordinary visit. It really requires some consideration and thought beforehand.

You will probably have to go some distance, spend some time and money, so you really want it to be a success, don't you? Too often ill people are left feeling bludgeoned, exhausted and defeated by their visitors, who go blithely on, quite unconscious of their blundering ways, indeed often delighted with themselves and their good deeds. This is why visiting is limited to certain hours and often to two persons at a time at the bedside. If, for any reason, you arrive at the hospital outside visiting hours, ask to see the sister of the ward – don't just try to barge in. The sister has a shrewd knowledge of people and will allow you in if she decides it is for her patient's benefit.

Conversation

You are going to limit your time at the bedside to about ten to twenty minutes, so you want everything you say to be of real value to the patient. If the weather is bad 'you are so lucky to be here' is not a helpful remark to someone who has just learned he has cancer or has lost a leg. He would willingly go out in any weather rather than find himself in his present circumstances. Use your imagination.

When you ask how the patient is, really listen to the reply. Let him talk about some aspect of his illness if he wishes, so that he can get it out of his system and so forget it. Try just to sit there and absorb whatever the patient wants to say. If he doesn't want to talk about his illness, don't pump him with questions. Your opinion is of no real value to him, so don't give it. Certainly don't tell him stories of friends of yours who either recovered in record time, or died of the same illness. Yes, I have had both experiences. In the first case I was made to feel guilty that it was my fault that I wasn't better. In the second I would have felt defeated, except that I found it funny that anyone could be so silly.

Long-winded accounts of your family and friends are difficult to follow, tiring and of little interest. Try to remain sensitive to the patient's need of the moment. If you can see even a glint of humour in the eye, a good laugh is the best medicine, but never try to impose heartiness on a person who is already weak and vulnerable. And don't hesitate as you leave. Do remember the patient is pinned to his bed, and can't help you through the door as he would in his own home. When you have stayed your ten to twenty minutes, get up, move to the door and *then go through it*. Don't stand talking so that the patient has to crick his neck looking up at you. This is exhausting. Of course an intimate relation or friend may stay a long time with good effect, but don't feel you have to be continually entertaining. Just sitting quietly can be a great comfort. Do stay with the unconscious. They may well be aware of your presence and find it helpful.

Presents and Flowers

First of all there is no need to take anything. What the

patient needs is diversion and gentleness not bundles of goods. If you are sending flowers keep them simple, if possible ready arranged in a disposable container. Shop roses droop their heads, try garden ones with buds to come out. Carnations and pinks last splendidly and give no trouble at any season, but don't include maidenhair fern which drops green particles continuously into everything including drinking water. Pieces of other green are excellent; they support the flowers and last well without dropping bits.

In winter a treat is a few paper-white narcissi, or daffodils in tight buds. In summer try a mixed posy of garden flowers – something from the daisy family last well, irises and gladioli can be entertaining as they gradually open. Beware of liles, they frighten some people who connect them with death, and of course there is the old hospital myth that red and white flowers together mean a death, so never use this mixture. One single orchid is wonderful, and is not necessarily as expensive as a bunch of flowers that will wilt in half the time. Often flower shops sell them all ready fixed in a tiny little sealed glass vase that can easily sit on the locker close to the eyes of the patient. It fulfils all the necessities of a good gift – colour, texture, unusual, exciting and yet completely devoid of any trouble to staff or patient. If you can possibly arrange for your flowers to await the arrival of the patient in hospital, that is best of all and most cheering.

Of course you never take anything to eat that the patient is not allowed. It isn't clever to try to break a special diet. It is cruel. Something exotic to eat is always a success, but again it must be carefully chosen, easy to eat and *small*. Your patient may prefer a little jar of jellied eels or a small smoked salmon sandwich. If anything needs a spoon or fork, then take that too. Grapes really are the best fruit, or a couple of bananas. Not any of the orange or tangerine tribe: they make the fingers smell. Not apples: they smell of themselves – a sickly, heavy smell in a closed ward. The Modern hospital has no open windows at all, only air conditioned, i.e. dry, air. Any smell you import is immediately intensified.

Try something home-made if you are a good cook, but keep it simple and plain. Chocolate melts, cream goes squashy. Anything incorporating fruit is refreshing, or what about a little pot of home-made jam or mayonnaise?

A small pretty salt and pepper set full of each is useful – both are elusive in hospital. A bottle of concentrated lemon juice or salad dressing is helpful; a china mug is heaven to drink out of, instead of the continuous paper cups. Air freshener and paper hankies in a pretty box make delightful presents. Give it some thought.

Convalescence is the time for carefully chosen books, crossword or jigsaw puzzles, patience cards, a small piece of knitting or embroidery, some seeds to sow.

The final present to help the person back to normal, is your time to take them out when they are home. You might help them in a neglected garden or with cooking or rearranging the house. Don't just forget them at what is often a very depressing time.

CONVALESCENCE

This is rather an uncomfortable no man's land. You are neither ill nor well, you are having rather less attention paid to your welfare, and you probably feel dreadful at times. It is possible that you sometimes feel that not only you, but also those who look after you are getting rather bored with the whole situation.

Try to take a day at a time and upgrade everything you can a little everyday. You must eat and drink sufficiently and you must sleep. Fresh air and some form of exercise are also essential to recovery. I suggest you look after these yourself, and so take the burden off the people attending to you who have probably had the tiring business of your real illness to bear. It is an enormous relief to them, for example, if you make up your mind what you would like to eat each day and ask for it, instead of always needing to be tempted to eat.

You must take the trouble every day to wash all over, get fully dressed, wear proper shoes, and brush your hair. This is a great morale booster for everyone and helps conquer irritability.

Remember the planar reflex (p. 76). Press your feet down firmly, stretch up your spine and head and get outside your front door every day, even for only a few minutes at the beginning. You might do your deep breathing in the fresh air. This is the time to begin some aerobic exercises (p. 84). Ask your doctor for permission. This means exercise using the larger groups of muscles that need a good supply of oxygen so that demands are made on your heart and lung system thus making those more efficient. You can begin gently. Try sitting, raising both your arms above your head quickly and continuously. Then you might try kicking alternate legs forward for a minute; or standing marking time raising your knees as high as possible. Never more than a minute at a time – just enough to make you a little breathless. In this way you may graduate to strong aerobic exercise when you are recovered.

Going downstairs can be very frightening especially if your balance is disturbed. Try going down backwards holding onto a rail with one hand and, if necessary, a stick in the other. You can even have someone behind you supporting your waist. Then you are absolutely safe. As you get stronger get rid of all these entanglements.

Getting better is seldom a continuous gradual improvement. It usually comes noticeably for a few days then either there is a setback, or you may stay the same for several days before another improvement. So don't expect too much too soon. Just keep at it.

GETTING BACK TO NORMAL

Getting back to normal is a step that some people just never achieve. They find it too difficult to come out of the nest of convalescence, where so much is done for them. I have spent my life looking after ill people, but I never realised, till it happened to me, just how complicated this phase is, and why many people find it too difficult to manage.

I had to relearn so much after years of making lists of shopping for others to do, of saying continuously 'Do you mind doing so and so'. But gradually I realised the relief of not having to ask any more. I could do the shopping, the washing, the cleaning, answer the phone and letters – and of course deal with what pain and disability still remained of the illness. This is all remarkably difficult at first.

Make the highlights – like the day they come to take away the wheelchair – the last call of the district nurse – a real celebration. Ask someone in for an easy meal and cook it yourself. Then make a list of all the friends who helped you when you were really ill, and gradually entertain each one. Make it their day with any discussion of your health now definitely barred. You have returned to normal, but it is a different normal from before you were ill. What you took for granted then, you now have to think about, and plan, and you will have a lot of failures. For example you overestimate your strength, do too much one day, and have to stay in bed all the next day to recover. Don't let this put you off. You are not going to remain a semi-invalid for the rest of your life. Be absolutely determined about that. You are creating a new kind of life for yourself, and it should be a fuller, happier one, because you will have learned a lot about yourself and other people.

Is it time, perhaps, for you to try to begin the long road of 'getting back to normal'? It may only be making a cup of tea for someone else instead of them making it for you, but that will do as a beginning.

Remember our mental, emotional and physical health is seldom static. It is either getting better or worse; be sure yours is on the upgrade, and think, in the words of the song, 'What a wonderful world'.

Book List

Books on Ageing and Health

Agate, J. *Taking Care of Old People at Home*, Allen & Unwin 1979

Burkitt, A. *Life Begins at Forty*, Health Education Council 1977

Carruthers, M. and Murray, A. *Fitness on Forty Minutes a Week*, Futura 1976

Centre for Policy on Ageing, *Keeping the Elderly Moving in Old People's Homes*, C.P.A. London 1981

Comfort, A. *A Good Age*, Mitchell Beazley 1977

Davison, W. *Stress in the Elderly*, Physiotherapy, April 1978, vol 64, no. 4

Dowson, J. *Fit for Living*, ITV Books

Eyton, A. *F Plan Diet*, Penguin 1982

Fries, J. and Crapo, L. *Vitality and Ageing*, Freeman 1981

Gore, I. *Age and Vitality*, Allen & Unwin 1979

Gray, M. *Better Health in Retirement*, Age Concern 1982

Gray, M. and Wilcock, G. *Our Elders*, OUP 1981

Guntrip, H. *Your Mind and Your Health*, Allen & Unwin 1979

Hart, D. *Overcoming Arthritis*, Martin Dunitz

Help the Aged, *The Time of Your Life*, Health Education Council 1982

Hooker, S. *Caring for Elderly People*, Routledge & Kegan Paul 1981

Howell, T. *Our Advancing Years*, Phoenix 1953

Mitchell, L. *Simple Relaxation*, John Murray 1977

Mitchell, L. and Dale, B. *Simple Movement*, John Murray 1980

Murray, A. and Bettsworth, M. *Towards Total Health*, Batsford 1981

Nicholson, J. *Seven Ages*, Fontana 1980

Oram, C. *Going Well Over 60*, Sunday Times/World's Work Ltd 1979

Scott-Moncrief, J. *The Sixty Plus Book*, Arrow 1977

Stinson, D. and Lough, R. *Aquatics Recreation and Fitness in Water*, Harper Colophon 1973

Stoddard, A. *The Back: Relief from Pain*, Martin Dunitz 1979

Stott, M. *Ageing for Beginners*, Blackwell 1981

Taylor, E. *Fitness After Forty*, John Murray 1966

de Vries, H., with Hales, D. *Fitness After 50*, Scribner, New York

Books on Pastimes and for Stimulus

Adams, M. *Natural Flower Arranging*, Batsford 1981

Berne, E. *Games People Play*, Penguin 1970

de Bono, E. *de Bono's Thinking Course*, BBC 1982

Bronowski, J. *The Ascent of Man*, BBC 1973

Bryant, C. *Jung and the Christian Way*, Darton Longman & Todd 1983

Churchill, Sir W.S. *Painting as a Pastime*, Odhams 1948

Clark, K. *Civilisation*, John Murray/BBC 1969

Clark, K. *Looking at Pictures*, John Murray 1960

Fermor, P. Leigh. *A Time to Keep Silence*, John Murray 1957

Harris, C.C. *House Plants*, Octopus 1979

Kempner, B. (Ed) *Macramé for Beginners*, Lyric Pattern Services 1979

Kimmond, J. *Teach Yourself Crochet*, Hodder & Stoughton 1979

Lees-Milne, A. and Verey, R. (Ed) *The Englishwoman's Garden*, Chatto & Windus 1980

Murray, L. *Michelangelo*, Thames & Hudson 1980

Nottingham, P. *Technique of Bobbin Lace*, Batsford 1976

Patten, M. *Bedsitter Cookery*, Hamlyn 1970

Smith, M.J. *When I Say No I Feel Guilty*, Bantam 1976

Southwell, S. *Painting China and Porcelain*, Blandford 1980

Index